HEALTH LITERACY IN A
NUTSHELL

Don Nutbeam | Danielle Muscat

HEALTH LITERACY IN A

NUTSHELL

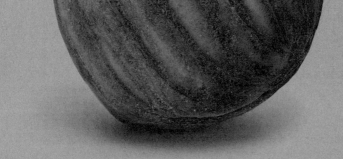

A practical guide to health communication

McGraw Hill

First edition published 2023

Text © 2023 Don Nutbeam & Danielle Muscat

Illustrations and design © 2023 McGraw Hill Education (Australia) Pty Ltd

Additional owners of copyright are acknowledged in on-page credits/on the acknowledgments page. Every effort has been made to trace and acknowledge copyrighted material. The authors and publishers tender their apologies should any infringement have occurred.

National Library of Australia Cataloguing-in-Publication Data:

A catalogue record for this book is available from the National Library of Australia

Authors: Don Nutbeam, Danielle Muscat
Title: Health Literacy in a Nutshell: a practical guide to health communication
Edition: 1st edition
ISBN: 9781760427337

Published in Australia by
McGraw Hill Education (Australia) Pty Ltd
Level 33, 680 George Street, Sydney NSW 2000
Publisher: Rochelle Deighton
Production manager: Martina Vascotto
Copyeditor: Julie Wicks
Proofreader: Meredith Lewin
Permissions manager: Rachel Norton
Cover and internal design: Simon Rattray, Squirt Creative
Cover image: Tiercel Studio/Shutterstock
Typeset by Straive
Printed in Singapore by Markono Print Media Pte Ltd

contents

list of tables, figures and case studies

TABLES

FIGURES

CASE STUDIES

preface

Health Literacy in a Nutshell is for students and frontline practitioners who want to improve their understanding of health literacy and to be better at health communication. Health education and public communication campaigns have always been an essential element of public health interventions and an important tool for prevention and health promotion. In the clinic, patient education has evolved considerably over past decades as patients and consumers have become essential partners in healthcare.

We know from practical experience that not everyone responds in the same way and with equal success to our health communications. There are many reasons why this is the case. Our communication methods may not be as good as we would wish and the media we use may not fit with individual preferences and patterns of media use. People can find the systems we operate within to be complex and confusing, especially in healthcare. The medical language we use routinely can be intimidating and alienating. We also know that people vary considerably in their skills, capacity and motivation to respond to our communications, and this can be compounded by the social and economic conditions that people experience.

Health Literacy in a Nutshell will help you understand how to be a better communicator and how to work more effectively with individuals and communities in helping them to find, understand, appraise and apply health information. It does so by exploring the concept of *health literacy* from multiple perspectives, beginning with a chapter exploring the concept and definition of health literacy. This is followed by chapters examining practical methods for working with patients, communities and organisations to improve health communications in ways that support people to take practical actions to improve and protect their health. The book also provides useful advice on the best ways to make use of digital media for health communication and for improving eHealth literacy, concluding with a chapter on health literacy, equity and the social determinants of health.

Health Literacy in a Nutshell provides pragmatic advice and guidance. It draws upon the best available scientific evidence and provides numerous practical examples of effective communication to improve health literacy among our patient and community populations. Each chapter includes helpful case studies, key references and advice on further reading. Even for experienced researchers and practitioners, the book provides a useful prompt on key issues, as well as guidance on how to organise and deliver interventions to improve health literacy.

about the authors

Don Nutbeam is a Professor of Public Health at the University of Sydney. His career has spanned senior leadership positions in universities, government, health services and international organisations, including the World Health Organization and the World Bank. He has research interests in the social and behavioural determinants of health, and in the development and evaluation of public health interventions.

Danielle Muscat is a Senior Research Fellow in the Sydney Health Literacy Lab at the University of Sydney and an Advisor on Health Literacy to the World Health Organization. With a passion for promoting equity, her research primarily focuses on the development and evaluation of interventions to improve health literacy among socially disadvantaged groups in both community and clinical settings.

1

Health literacy concepts and definitions

1.1 Introduction

So much of what we do in healthcare and public health relies upon people being engaged in decisions about their health. Health education and public communication campaigns have always been an essential element of public health. In the clinic, patient education has evolved over past decades as people have become partners in decisions about their healthcare. We know from practical experience that not everyone responds in the same way and with equal success to our health communications. There are many reasons why this is the case—our communication methods may not be as good as we would wish; individuals vary considerably in their skills, capacity and motivation to respond to them; and the social and economic conditions that people experience may not support the response we are hoping for.

This book is intended to help you understand how to be a better communicator and how to work more effectively with individuals and communities in helping them to find, understand, appraise and apply health information. It will do so by exploring the concept of *health literacy* from multiple perspectives.

1.2 Literacy, language and health literacy

Literacy has been defined as *"the ability to understand, evaluate, use, and engage with written texts to participate in society, achieve one's goals, and develop one's knowledge and potential"* (OECD, 2013). This definition makes clear why societies around the world place great value on achieving high levels of literacy in their populations. It focuses attention on what literacy helps us to achieve—enabling people to better develop their knowledge and improve their potential to achieve personal goals. Higher levels of literacy also enable individuals to participate more fully in society and the economy.

Literacy is also associated both directly and indirectly with a range of health outcomes. Low literacy is often associated with established social determinants of health, including, for example, employment status and lifetime income. We also know that people with poor literacy also tend to be less responsive to traditional health education messages, are less likely to use disease prevention services and are less able to successfully manage illness.

Fortunately, literacy is not a fixed asset. It can be improved, especially through formal education and through structured communication. People can develop their literacy skills from basic, word level skills (such as recognising words) through to higher level skills (such as understanding and analysing meaning from continuous text). Individuals vary in their ability to learn and will respond in diverse ways to the stimulus provided by different forms of communication and media. Each of these issues is examined critically throughout this book.

Literacy should not be confused with language spoken. This is especially important in multicultural populations where many people in communities speak a language other than English. In populations where English may be a second or third language, it is important not to confuse the ability to respond to a communication because of low literacy with the ability to respond because of poor English language skills. A person may be highly literate in their chosen language but at a disadvantage in understanding communications in English. In these circumstances, improving communication may depend fundamentally on making information available in languages other than English, and recognising different cultural preferences in content and communication method. Some individuals may also have low literacy in their chosen language, which further compounds the task of communication. As we will discuss later in the book, it is important to take into account both literacy and language in managing successful communication.

The possession of generic literacy skills in reading, writing and understanding text (as well as related numeracy skills) greatly enhances the ability of an individual to find, understand and act on all forms of new information. However, having these literacy skills provides no guarantee that a person can consistently apply them in situations that require specific content knowledge or that place a person in an unfamiliar setting. For example, even a person with high literacy skills may experience real challenges in applying these skills in an unfamiliar environment (like a hospital or when online) or in interacting with a person (like a health professional) that they find unfamiliar and intimidating. In short, everyone has varying capacity to apply their general literacy skills in different contexts.

Literacy can thus be viewed as context specific. It can be understood as the application of personal literacy skills that are mediated by the environment in which these skills are to be applied. *Health literacy* can be viewed within this framework as a specific form of literacy that is shaped both by the personal skills necessary for the acquisition of health-related knowledge, and the context in which this knowledge is to be applied.

1.3 Defining health literacy

Numerous definitions of health literacy have been proposed. Figure 1.1 provides a widely used framework that makes explicit the extent to which a person's health literacy skills are mediated by the situational demands and complexities that are placed on people. If health literacy is understood as an observable set of personal skills, this necessarily focuses our attention on improving individuals' skills and capacities through communication and education. Recognising the demands and complexities of different situations/contexts also focuses attention on simplifying communication and reducing organisational complexities. Both represent important methods for addressing the challenges posed by poor health literacy in the health system and in the wider community.

Given this background and context, health literacy is defined as follows:

> *Health literacy represents the personal competencies and organizational structures, resources and commitment which enable people to access, understand, appraise and use information and services in ways which promote and maintain good health.*

This is adapted from the formal World Health Organization (WHO) definition originally developed by the authors (Nutbeam & Muscat, 2021), and explicitly reflects both personal and situational elements in Figure 1.1. The WHO definition provides further explanation: "Health literacy is founded on inclusive and equitable access to quality education and life-long learning. The definition emphasises that health literacy is not the sole responsibility

Figure 1.1 Health literacy: Enhancing personal skills and reducing system complexity

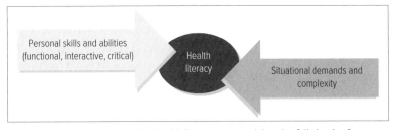

Adapted from: Parker R, Ratzan SC. Health literacy: a second decade of distinction for Americans. J Health Commun. 2010;15 Suppl 2:20-33. Reprinted by permission of the publisher (Taylor &Francis Ltd, http://www.tandfonline.com)

of individuals. All information providers, including government, civil society and health services, should enable access to trustworthy information in a form that is understandable and actionable for all people."

This definition of health literacy also makes explicit that "health literacy means more than being able to access websites, read pamphlets and follow prescribed behaviours. It includes the ability to exercise critical judgement of health information and resources, as well as the ability to interact and express personal and societal needs for promoting health". These important concepts of interacting with information and those who provide it and of critical judgement are examined further below.

Poor health literacy is very common in all populations. Most national and international studies of adult health literacy have identified that a majority in the population have "inadequate" health literacy. This means that only a minority in the adult population have the literacy skills to manage even some of the most basic challenges of finding trustworthy information, interpreting advice and instructions, and in navigating the healthcare system. There is much we can do to help people develop their health literacy skills and confidence and the onus is on us all to improve the quality of our communications, to find the most interactive ways to engage with our patients and community members, and to reduce the numerous access barriers to reliable, understandable health information in all environments (healthcare, community, online).

1.4   Functional, interactive and critical health literacy

As is the case in general literacy, health literacy represents an observable set of skills that will vary from individual to individual. These differences in personal skills have been categorised as *functional, interactive* and *critical health literacy*. Such a classification has the advantage of helping us understand better the impact that differences in skill levels may have on health-related decisions and actions, and in the responsiveness of individuals to different forms of health communication and education.

Functional health literacy describes basic-level skills that are sufficient for individuals to obtain relevant health information (for example, on health risks and on how to use the health system), and to be able to apply that knowledge to a range of well-defined actions. Individuals with these basic health literacy skills are generally able to respond well to education and communication that is directed to clearly defined goals within a specific context. This might include understanding correct dosage of medications; participation in prevention activities such as screening and immunisation programs; and engaging in behavioural change (such as quitting smoking, changing diet or increasing physical activity).

Interactive health literacy describes more advanced literacy skills that incrementally build on those described above to enable people to actively extract health information and derive meaning from different forms of communication; to apply new information to changing circumstances; and to engage in interactions with others to extend the information available and make decisions. Individuals with these higher level skills are better able to discriminate between different sources of information; to respond to health communication and education that is more interactive and accessible through structured communication channels (for example, school health education, mobile apps and interactive websites); and to adapt their responses to health information to reflect this deeper understanding.

Critical health literacy describes the most advanced literacy skills that incrementally build on those described above to enable people to critically analyse information from a wide range of sources and on a greater range of health determinants. This will include information appraisal both on personal health risks and on the social, economic and environmental determinants of health. Individuals with these most advanced skills can obtain and use information to exert greater control over life events and situations that have an impact on health. This not only includes the type of adaptive change described above, but also using information for negotiation, collective organising and action. This type of health literacy can be more obviously linked to population benefit alongside benefits to the individual.

The concept of functional health literacy aligns more closely to the immediate and necessary goals of clinical care and some public health priorities. For example, health literacy may be seen as a relatively stable patient characteristic—a *risk* that needs to be managed in the process of providing clinical care. The implications of this are that clinicians need to modify their communication with patients as a *universal precaution* in anticipation of lower levels of health literacy, and where possible, reduce the organisational demands and complexity faced by patients in a clinical environment. Reducing complexity might include simplifying appointment procedures and communications about them, and reducing the complexity and use of jargon in written patient information and advice. We discuss the practice of universal health literacy precautions further in Chapter 2, and provide advice on simplifying written and online communications in Chapters 2 and 4.

In many clinical situations, people often need the most basic knowledge and functional skills required to follow healthcare instructions and guidance that are primarily determined by those providing healthcare. Community health education can also be similarly task-based and goal-directed—promoting improved knowledge for specific behaviour changes and expecting those receiving the communication to respond.

The concepts of interactive and critical health literacy align more closely to contemporary approaches to health promotion and consumer involvement in healthcare. In this case, improving health literacy helps develop the personal skills and confidence that support greater engagement, more autonomy and better control over health decision-making. Working with people to develop transferable health literacy skills that can be applied in a wide variety of circumstances necessitates a fundamentally different approach to health communication in both methods and content. It requires the use of more interactive and adaptable communication methods, such as to incorporate consumer preferences, enable development of skills in shared decision-making and prompt critical evaluation of information content and sources. More advanced, critical health literacy skills would be reflected in substantial knowledge of the social determinants of health and skills in negotiation, social mobilisation and consumer advocacy. This is in marked contrast to many established communication models based on changing specific knowledge, attitudes and behaviours. While goal-directed communication will always have a place in health and patient education, re-thinking health communication as a vehicle for improving transferable health literacy skills in this way can have a transformative influence on the purpose and methodologies of modern health education and patient education. This fundamental challenge in health communication is discussed further throughout the book.

It is also important to recognise that both content and context change through the life-course. Thus, for example, the health literacy skills and content for decision-making needed by an adolescent in navigating decisions about the use of alcohol with their peer group differ markedly from the knowledge and skills needed by a couple expecting their first child, or a person diagnosed with diabetes in middle age. The actions necessary to improve health literacy and reduce the complexity of communications will vary accordingly.

Although our school system has an important role in providing foundational health knowledge and literacy skills, health literacy is not something established at one time and for all time through formal education. Because it is content and context specific, we need to be constantly aware of the challenges that individuals face throughout the life-course in *accessing, understanding, appraising and using information in ways which promote and maintain good health.* We refer to the different challenges faced by individuals and ways of addressing them throughout the following chapters.

1.5 Improving health literacy

Considerable attention has been given to the definition and measurement of health literacy in different populations. This has highlighted the extent of the challenges associated with low health literacy and encourages us to think about different approaches to improving health literacy. In this book we consistently refer to four broad strategies for improving health literacy that have variable application in clinical and community settings. These are summarised in Figure 1.2.

Figure 1.2 offers a dynamic view of the different methods for improving health literacy. The two core aims highlight the need to develop personal skills and abilities (1) alongside action to reduce the situational demands and complexity (2) faced by people in accessing, appraising, understanding and using health information. Four strategies are highlighted for improving health literacy. Two are identified to help develop personal skills and abilities—improving access to accurate, trustworthy information across the life-course (3); and working directly with the public and patients to develop skills and confidence in applying information (4) in ways that promote and protect health. Two further strategies are identified to help reduce situational demands and complexities—reducing the complexity/improving the quality of communication with patients and the public (5); and regulating the information environment (6) in ways that make it easier to access accurate and trustworthy health information.

Figure 1.2 also highlights some of the connections between the different strategies, illustrating, for example, the fundamental importance of improving the quality of communications in order to widen access (7) and optimise authentic consumer engagement with health information (8); and the role of health professionals and consumer groups in advocating for better regulation

Figure 1.2 Improving health literacy

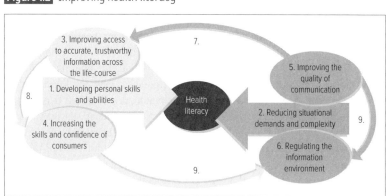

of the health information environment (9). Each of these strategies is considered further in the following chapters.

These aims and strategies are not intended to be mutually exclusive. They can operate separately and concurrently at different levels, working with individuals, communities, organisations and through public policy. Choosing the "right" approach will always be moderated by the practical opportunities for action. Those working with individual patients or in communities at a local level need to use local knowledge and experience, as well as available research information, to make judgments about patient/community needs that are most amenable to intervention. This might include understanding how to best connect with those that work with these communities, such as multicultural health workers. Not all of us have capacity to operate at multiple levels, but a knowledge of these strategies can help us to maximise the potential effectiveness of the opportunities we have and place them in a broader context.

1.6   Summary

Health literacy is content and context specific: Health literacy has evolved as a distinctive concept over the past 25 years. It is a specific form of literacy that is shaped both by the personal skills necessary for the acquisition of health-related knowledge, and the context in which this knowledge is to be applied. Health literacy is defined formally as: *"the personal competencies and organizational structures, resources and commitment which enable people to access, understand, appraise and use information and services in ways which promote and maintain good health".*

More advanced health literacy skills include the ability to exercise critical judgment of health information and resources, as well as the ability to interact and express personal and societal needs for promoting health.

Most people experience difficulty in finding and using health information: National studies have revealed that a significant proportion of the population have difficulty in accessing, understanding, appraising and using health information. Only a minority in the adult population have the literacy skills to manage even some of the most basic challenges of finding trustworthy information, interpreting advice and instructions, and in navigating the healthcare system. These challenges are exacerbated by a lack of effective communication, ineffective choices of media that are not nuanced or tailored to community population needs, and unnecessarily complicated interactions with health organisations and health professionals.

Health literacy can be improved. There is much we can do to help people develop their health literacy skills and confidence, and the onus is on us all to improve the quality of our communications; to find the most interactive ways to engage with our patients and community members; and to reduce the numerous access barriers to reliable, understandable health information in all environments (healthcare, community, online). This requires carefully tailored communication and media selection and, increasingly, a better regulated information environment.

References

Nutbeam D, Muscat DM 2021. Health Promotion Glossary 2021. *Health Promotion International,* 36(6), 1578-1598. doi: 10.1093/heapro/daaa157

OECD (Organisation for Economic Co-operation and Development) 2013. Skilled for Life? Key findings from the survey of adult skills. Available from: https://www.oecd.org/skills/piaac/SkillsOutlook_2013_ebook.pdf

Parker R, Ratzan S 2010. Health literacy: a second decade of distinction for Americans. *Journal of Health Communication,* 15(2), 20–33. doi: 10.1080/10810730.2010.501094

Further reading

Berkman ND, Sheridan SL, Donahue KE, Halpern DJ, Crotty K 2011. Low health literacy and health outcomes: an updated systematic review. *Annals of Internal Medicine,* 155(2), 97–107. doi:10.7326/0003-4819-155-2-201107190-00005

Nutbeam D 2000. Health literacy as a public health goal: a challenge for contemporary health education and communication strategies into the 21st century. *Health Promotion International,* 15(3), 259–267. doi:10.1093/heapro/15.3.259

Nutbeam D 2008. The evolving concept of health literacy. *Social Science & Medicine,* 67(12), 2072–2078. doi:10.1016/j.socscimed.2008.09.050

Sørensen K, Van den Broucke S, Fullam J, Doyle G, Pelikan J, et al. 2012. Health literacy and public health: a systematic review and integration of definitions and models. *BMC Public Health,* 12(1), 80. doi:10.1186/1471-2458-12-80

2

Improving health literacy in clinical settings: health literacy for frontline health workers

2.1 Introduction

Frontline health workers are regularly identified by the public as the most highly trusted sources of health information. As such, we have a corresponding responsibility to provide health information that is both accurate and tailored to the needs of our patients and consumers. Many government agencies and health-related civil society organisations (heart foundations, cancer organisations, etc.) enjoy the same level of trust and have the same responsibilities.

Disappointingly, research has demonstrated that we consistently fail to communicate effectively to our patients, consumers and communities. This applies in all settings—face-to-face in the clinic, online through different digital platforms and in the wider community through different media and networks. We use words that are medically correct but alienating for most people; we use language that is complex and often beyond the literacy and language skills of our consumers; and especially in clinical locations, we fail to mitigate the stressful environment in which people are receiving complex health advice. By contrast, opportunities to help individuals to become more engaged and autonomous in health decision-making are frequently missed as we place emphasis on "compliance" and encourage passivity in the methods and content of our communication.

No one intends it to be this way and the reasons why we come up short are often complex, especially in a pressured, time poor, dynamic clinical environment. Fortunately, we now have a more sophisticated understanding of effective communication methods, underpinned by research and practical experience. This body of knowledge has helped identify a range of evidence-based strategies for improving written and verbal health communication that are practical to implement even in busy clinical environments. This chapter provides an overview of principles and practical tools for effective communication with an emphasis on their application in clinical settings.

2.2 Universal precautions

In Chapter 1, we identified that a majority of the population in most countries have difficulty in understanding even basic health information, and that this difficulty is exacerbated in a clinical environment. Past research has indicated that most information exchanged during a medical consultation is either forgotten immediately or recalled incorrectly. For these reasons, it is generally recommended that frontline practitioners use *health literacy universal precautions*. This simply means that we should assume that all patients, consumers and caregivers may have difficulty in comprehending health information; and that we should communicate in ways that most people can understand. This approach, pioneered and advocated by the US Agency for Healthcare Research and Quality, assumes that all patients are at risk for miscommunication and misunderstanding, regardless of education, socioeconomic status or literacy skills. A universal precautions approach is based on research that has identified limited health literacy is common and that patients may go to great lengths to conceal their lack of understanding, that frontline health professionals are insufficiently skilled at detecting when patients do not understand and that formal assessment of a patient's health literacy in clinical settings is unrealistic.

The application of health literacy universal precautions recognises the practical realities faced by many frontline health professionals in normal clinical conditions. It is based on research and practical experience indicating that even the most highly educated/highly literate individuals can find that the stresses of the clinical environment overwhelm their ability to absorb information and understand advice. Related research has identified that more highly educated individuals welcome health information that is simplified and thoughtfully communicated. The practical challenge is to find communication methods and tools that make this feasible in routine practice. We examine key methods that have been shown to have greatest potential below.

2.3 Effective person-to-person communication

Teach-back

Teach-back is a health communication strategy used to confirm patient understanding in a non-judgemental way. It has been successfully used in a wide range of environments in which person-to-person communication may occur, including hospital and clinic settings as well as consumer telephone helplines. Teach-back builds on basic concepts of active listening and respectful communication. It simply involves asking patients and consumers to explain in their own words what a frontline health worker has just told them.

This simple technique will quickly identify any confusion or misunderstanding and provide the basis for further clarification. Following clarification, patients are asked again to explain the advice in their own words and the process continues until the patient can recall the key points communicated with reasonable understanding. Critical in this process is the assurance to patients that they are not being "tested", and that the purpose of the request is to check that the frontline professional has been successful with their communication. The onus for a successful outcome is not on the understanding of the patient, but on the communication skills of the health provider.

The 'e' model shown in Figure 2.1 illustrates the steps involved in Teachback. As a first step, it is the responsibility of the health professional to use simplified language to provide essential health information to patients. (1). The next step is to evaluate the success of communication by asking the patient to repeat that information in their own words (to teach-back) (2). If patients cannot repeat back the information provided (or do so incorrectly), it is responsibility of the health professional to identify miscommunication, explain and improve communication as necessary (3). Continue through the 'e' loop until the patient can accurately communicate in their own words (4), at which stage the communication can end and the patient should be empowered to manage their health (5).

Using Teach-back for the first time can be quite confronting for healthcare providers who discover just how little of their communication has been

Figure 2.1 The teachback 'e'

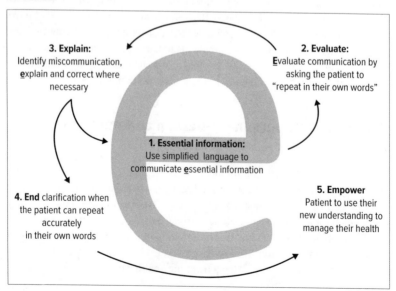

understood by a patient or caregiver. But it is a proven, effective way of gaining real-time feedback on communication and provides clear targets for improved communication. Practice supports continuous improvement. The extra time taken to get the communication right will improve both learning-related outcomes (e.g. knowledge recall and retention) as well as objective health-related outcomes (e.g. hospital re-admissions, quality of life). The proficiency of using the Teach-back approach will improve each time with use, and time taken with each patient will reduce with experience.

Shared decision-making

Teach-back is an excellent technique to improve patient knowledge and understanding. It can also help to develop patient skills and confidence in health decision-making as they become more familiar with the issues and more experienced in interacting with healthcare professionals. In clinical practice it is increasingly important for patients to be more actively involved both in making decisions about options for care and in managing continuing illness. This involves health provider communication and consumer engagement that fits more obviously with the concept of interactive health literacy described in Chapter 1.

One of the best researched and commonly used methods for achieving more meaningful consumer engagement is shared decision-making. Shared decision-making involves discussion and collaboration between a consumer and their healthcare provider. It is defined as a process of bringing together a consumer's values, goals and preferences with the best available evidence about benefits, risks and uncertainties of different treatment options in order to reach the best possible healthcare decision for that person. Critical in this definition is the commitment to using best available evidence tempered by respect for patients' values and preferences.

Shared decision-making recognises the autonomy and responsibility of both health professionals *and* patients. However, making decisions in this way may be unfamiliar for many patients, who often feel that they cannot or should not be involved in decisions, who may not be aware that they have a choice and who often expect the clinician to tell them what treatment they "need". Such views and beliefs are deeply engrained in many patients, and often form a part of their cultural beliefs and respect for authority.

To address such barriers, shared decision-making interventions are best delivered in two stages: *preparation,* followed by *enablement* (Joseph-Williams, et al., 2014). First, patients should be provided with a *preparation* intervention, such as a booklet and/or website link, with their appointment letter. This type of communication should:

- inform patients about shared decision-making—what it is, what to expect and why it is important for their healthcare

- explain that there are two experts in the clinical encounter—the clinician and the patient—each with different but complementary knowledge
- reassure patients that there are no inherently right and wrong decisions
- redefine perceptions of a good patient and reassure patients that participation will not result in adverse consequences
- promote social acceptability of this role—confirm that clinicians want patient participation
- build patients' belief in their ability to take part.

Once the patient has made an informed decision to be involved, the focus moves on to *enablement*. This is helping patients to take part in the shared decision-making process by offering relevant and useful decision support tools, such as a patient decision aid. At a minimum, a decision aid describes the decision to be taken, the options available and the outcomes of these options (including benefits, harms and uncertainties) based on a careful review of the evidence. An inventory of decision aids can be found online at: https://decisionaid.ohri.ca/AZlist.html.

It is important that decision aids include clear, easy-to-understand information about the condition and the treatment or support options. This can be achieved by calculating readability scores, simplifying text and using graphics, animations and other techniques to reduce cognitive effort, as well as by including patients of all literacy levels in the development process. These strategies are described in greater detail below. Alternative formats for decision support, such as Option Grids, have also been developed which generally have less textual information compared to typical decision aids and are designed to be used jointly by the patient and their healthcare provider during a consultation.

Patient decision aids are a relatively new tool for patient education and have not always been developed with lower literacy populations in mind. As a consequence, decision aids have often been limited in their reach and impact. Much closer attention needs to be given to simplifying information using the methods described. It is also necessary to remember that many patients will be unfamiliar and culturally uncomfortable with the concept of shared decision-making and will need to have their confidence and skills built up over time. While there are limitations on opportunities for patient education in clinical settings, there are excellent examples of structured patient education to support shared decision-making in the management of chronic and continuing illness. For example, the Chronic Disease Self-Management Program, a 6-week peer-led program for people living with chronic disease first developed by Stanford University, includes topics on "communication skills" and "making informed treatment decisions". By developing these adaptable skills, individuals with established chronic diseases are much better equipped to partner in the management of their disease and respond to the dynamic and evolving nature of their chronic condition.

Beyond the clinical environment, the underlying concept of shared decision-making has been extended into public health and community settings within interventions designed to improve health literacy; for example, in community prevention programs, adult education, antenatal and parenting education programs. These are discussed in greater detail in the following chapter.

2.4 Written communication and plain language

The time available for face-to-face verbal communication will always be limited in a clinical setting and many clinicians rely on additional, written health information to supplement their communication. This written information may be in the form of a pamphlet or other traditional media, but is increasingly accessible online and through mobile devices. Sadly, much of this written information uses medical jargon and complex language that seriously limits its usefulness for many patients and consumers. There are several tools and techniques that can be used to address this to ensure that written information is accessible and understandable to a much larger proportion of the population.

Readability

Assessing the readability of written health information is the most common way to evaluate whether or not it is likely to be easily understood by the majority of people for whom it is intended. Readability is a measure of reading ease. This is calculated using simple tools that examine the use of words and sentences (including, for example, the number of syllables per word and words per sentence) to estimate a readability score, usually in the form of a school grade reading level. Internationally, there are several literacy (and health literacy) policy documents that include recommendations for health information to be written at a certain grade reading level, usually grade 8 (age 13-14) or below. Unfortunately, the great majority of written information from clinical service providers has been found to be written at higher grade levels, often at levels that can only be easily understood by people with post-graduate level education!

There are several different readability formulas to help assess the complexity of written sentences. For example, the Simple Measure of Gobbledygook (SMOG) Index is based on assessment of the number of polysyllabic words, while the Flesch–Kincaid Grade Level (FKGL) is based on assessment of the number of words per sentence and of syllables per word. The Automated Readability Index (ARI), on the other hand, relies on the number of characters per word as well as the number of words per sentence.

The SMOG Index is often recommended for health communication because it has been validated against 100% comprehension. This means that people with a grade 8 reading ability would score 100% on a multiple-choice comprehension test for text written at a grade 8 level. On the other hand, the FKGL, which is often built into word processing software, only assumes 75% comprehension, and can underestimate the grade reading level by 2–3 grades.

There are now many readily available online calculators which provide readability estimates within seconds, including those providing SMOG and FKGL scores. Some also provide practical advice and tips on changes necessary to improve readability. Users are simply required to cut and paste their proposed text into a box and will receive feedback on reading age and potential improvements immediately.

One of these, the SHeLL Health Literacy Editor, is illustrated in Figure 2.2. The SHeLL Editor has been specifically designed to support the development

Figure 2.2 The Health Literacy Editor

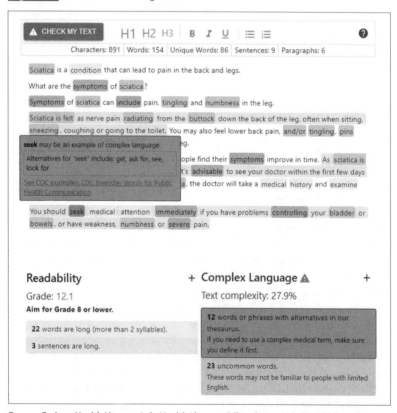

Source: Sydney Health Literacy Lab. Health Literacy Editor. https://shell.techlab.works/

of health-literate written health information (Ayre et al., 2023). It objectively assesses readability, complex language, passive voice, text structure, word density and diversity, and person-centred language. By explicitly aligning features with existing health literacy guidelines, the tool provides health information developers with a targeted tool to improve the quality and safety of health information. Assessments are provided in real-time, supporting iterative revisions to reduce text complexity. It complements the widely used readability scores referred to with other relevant assessments, including those specific to health.

With such digital technologies available to us there really is little excuse not to test and simplify the language used in all forms of written communication. Artificial intelligence (AI) apps and services are rapidly emerging and may also help to generate content, simplify text and edit language. The use of AI in health communication is a fast-developing field that offers great potential to further assist us in creating accessible and understandable health information.

Readability and translation

One drawback of readability assessments is the limited application to texts in non-English languages. So far, readability tools are only validated in English and select languages within the Indo-European language family. The Flesch–Kincaid Reading Ease and SMOG, for example, have been successfully applied to evaluate health materials in Spanish-language text after adjusting the increased average syllable count and sentence length in Spanish. However, materials written in other languages cannot be assessed using existing readability tools owing to different linguistic structures and rules. In such cases, health literacy guidelines often recommend using readability tools to assess source texts (a text to be used as a template for translation) with the view of simplifying medical terminology and jargon and streamlining the translation process. In this way, readability tools for English-language materials may still have practical value in assessing the health literacy demand of materials developed for culturally and linguistically diverse groups. Texts with lower grade reading scores in English generally support higher quality translations. As indicated in the previous section, there is also great potential for the application of AI tools and software in the simplification and translation of written health communication materials.

Other tools and resources

Readability is a convenient but relatively narrow assessment of the health literacy demand of materials. There are a number of other textual (e.g. use of active voice) and non-textual factors (e.g. use of visual aids) that influence reading comprehension. For this reason, the Health Literacy Universal Precautions Toolkit recommends using a range of methods to examine the quality of written materials. Here, we introduce several of these tools.

Each of these tools can be found using the AHRQ Health Literacy Universal Precautions Toolkit link in the further reading section of the references.

The Patient Education Materials Assessment Tool (PEMAT)

The PEMAT was developed by the Agency for Healthcare Research and Quality to assess the understandability and actionability of patient education materials, including both printable and audio-visual materials. The tools cover (1) content, (2) word style and choice, (3) use of numbers (4) organisation, (5) layout and design, and (6) the use of visuals, with higher scores indicating that health materials are easier to understand and act on. The PEMAT has recently been adapted to also evaluate the cultural appropriateness of health information (Abdi et al., 2020).

CDC Clear Communication Index

The Index contains 20 items, categorised into seven areas related to: (1) main message and call to action, (2) language, (3) information design, (4) state of the science, (5) behavioural recommendations, (6) numbers and (7) risk. Each item is assigned a numerical score of zero or one and individual scores are converted to an overall score on a scale of 100. Although 100 is an ideal score, 90 or higher is considered "passing".

Suitability Assessment of Materials (SAM)

The SAM instrument rates materials on factors that affect readability and comprehension in six areas: (1) content, (2) literacy demand, (3) graphics, (4) layout and type, (5) learning stimulation and motivation, and (6) cultural appropriateness. For each factor, materials are rated as Superior, Adequate or Not Suitable based on objective criteria included in the instrument, and an overall score and a score for each area can be calculated.

2.5 Consumer testing and co-design

One of the most obvious ways of improving the quality and safety of health information is to partner with patients, consumers, their families and carers when developing content and presentation. The benefits of consumer engagement and co-design are well documented within the broader health literature, showing improved outcomes for healthcare, service delivery, policy and health education. This can be done very formally through systematic, formative evaluation of materials and communication methods prior to their use. Such formative evaluation can range from a thorough review of existing examples (Is there already something that is effective and available? Can it be adapted for use in your clinic?), through to more formal pilot studies and evaluations working directly with your clinical population, local communities or other end-users of your service. While this may not be a practical solution for all written communications, checking-in with patients and consumers using a modified Teach-back methodology is a simple and quick way to test knowledge gain and understanding from a patient's use of written materials.

Co-design goes beyond the more traditional partnering methods, such as those described, because it enables consumers to become equal partners in health information development. They can often provide useful practical input to a range of written health communication materials that a clinician or manager may not have thought of as being useful or necessary. Fundamental to co-design is the equal status of clinicians and consumers in the design, testing and development of health communication materials. Such a partnership places high value on the lived experiences and cultural diversity of both health consumers and health professionals. Co-design is challenging for both patients and professionals but becoming more common in health service delivery as organisations and health professionals recognise the value of involving people with a lived experience of a relevant service or health condition.

This broader concept of co-design has been embraced in health literacy. One of the best-established methodologies is the Ophelia (OPtimising HEalth LIterAcy) protocol, which has been used successfully in a variety of settings in several countries. It involves investigating the health literacy strengths, needs and preferences of individuals and groups of people (for example, through the use of validated questionnaires) and drawing on local knowledge and wisdom alongside international evidence to co-design, develop and implement health literacy strategies that are accessible, sustainable and useful for the people who need them. The Ophelia protocol supports health workers in a systematic process of co-design with the population intended to benefit from a health literacy improvement program.

The Ophelia protocol has been applied and/or adapted for use in several countries around the world and found to be a practical tool for the successful engagement of clinical and community populations in the development of interventions. It has been designed to fit with the quality improvement programs of many health organisations. The co-design elements have been shown to generate locally relevant and fit-for-purpose interventions that are more easily implemented. This same research also demonstrated a range of important outcomes including organisational level process improvements,

Figure 2.3 Ophelia (OPtimising HEalth LIterAcy) phases

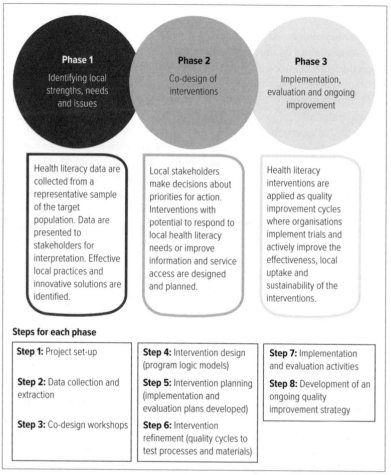

Source: Beauchamp, A., Batterham, R.W., Dodson, S. et al. Systematic development and implementation of interventions to OPtimise Health Literacy and Access (Ophelia). BMC Public Health 17, 230 (2017). https://doi.org/10.1186/s12889-017-4147-5.

improvements in staff knowledge and skills, improvements in community engagement and direct improvements in client outcomes and equity.

While not feasible to implement for every population in all circumstances, the Ophelia protocol can provide a well-structured process for considering how best to systematically incorporate consumer knowledge and preferences into interventions to improve health literacy with defined populations.

2.6 Summary

As trusted sources of health information we have a responsibility to get communication right: Frontline health workers, government agencies and civil society organisations are the most highly trusted sources of health information and have a responsibility to provide information that is accessible and tailored to the needs of patients and consumers. We frequently fall short of meeting consumers' needs by using language that is complex and often beyond their literacy and language skills, and fail to create an environment for communication that supports meaningful engagement and builds consumer confidence. There are a range of methodologies, tools and protocols that we can use to improve this situation.

Universal precautions are necessary: Because the risk of misunderstanding is so high among such a large proportion of our clinical populations, the use of health literacy universal precautions is advocated. This assumes that all patients are at risk for miscommunication and misunderstanding, regardless of education, socioeconomic status or literacy skills.

Effective communication techniques are available and convenient to use in clinical practice: Use of techniques such as Teach-back offer a relatively simple method for checking and improving patient understanding of health information in routine clinical practice. There are also simple, practical language editing tools to assist with the simplification of language and sentence construction when preparing written materials.

Patient engagement in clinical decision-making is feasible and leads to better outcomes: There is strong and consistent evidence that meaningful patient engagement in clinical decision-making leads to better health outcomes. There are practical methodologies and useful decision aids that can support clinicians who want to facilitate shared decision-making. These methodologies can enable patients to develop their health literacy skills to make better decisions and empower them in the management of their illness. While not realistic for all clinicians in all circumstances, evidence of the benefits of active consumer engagement in the co-development of communication methods and materials is strong.

References

Abdi I, Murphy B, Seale H 2020. Evaluating the health literacy demand and cultural appropriateness of online immunisation information available to refugee and migrant communities in Australia. *Vaccine,* 38(41), 6410–6417. doi:10.1016/j.vaccine.2020.07.071

Ayre J, Bonner C, Muscat D, Dunn A, Harrison E, et al. 2023. Multiple automated health literacy assessments of written health information: development of the SHeLL (Sydney Health Literacy Lab) Health Literacy Editor v1. *JMIR Formative Research,* 7: e40645. https:// formative.jmir.org/2023/1/e40645. doi: 10.2196/40645

Beauchamp A, Batterham RW, Dodson S, Astbury B, Elsworth GR, et al. 2017. Systematic development and implementation of interventions to OPtimise Health Literacy and Access (Ophelia). *BMC Public Health,* 17(1), 230. doi:10.1186/s12889-017-4147-5

Joseph-Williams N, Edwards A, Elwyn G 2014. Power imbalance prevents shared decision making. *BMJ,* 348, g3178–g3178. doi:10.1136/bmj.g3178

Sydney Health Literacy Lab. Health Literacy Editor. https://shell.techlab. works/

Further reading

AHRQ Health Literacy Universal Precautions Toolkit 2020. Agency for Healthcare Research and Quality, Rockville, MD. https://www.ahrq. gov/health-literacy/improve/precautions/index.html

Australian Commission on Safety and Quality in Healthcare 2022. *Shared decision making.* Sydney, Australia. https://www.safetyandquality.gov. au/our-work/partnering-consumers/shared-decision-making

British Medical Journal 2013. An introduction to patient decision aids. *BMJ,* 347(7918), 27–29. doi:10.1136/bmj.f4147

DeWalt DA, Broucksou KA, Hawk V, Brach C, Hink A, et al. 2011. Developing and testing the health literacy universal precautions toolkit. *Nursing Outlook,* 59(2), 85–94. doi:10.1016/j.outlook.2010.12.002

Muscat DM, Smith J, Mac O, Cadet T, Giguere A, et al. 2021. Addressing health literacy in patient decision aids: an update from the International Patient Decision Aid Standards. *Medical Decision Making,* 41(7), 848–869. doi:10.1177/0272989X211011101

Peters P, Liao S, Kruger J-L, Orlando M 2022. *Effective public messaging in online communication for all Australians.* Macquarie University, Sydney, Australia. https://researchers.mq.edu.au/en/publications/effective-public-messaging-in-online-communication-for-all-austra

Talevski J, Wong Shee A, Rasmussen B, Kemp G, Beauchamp A 2020. Teach-back: a systematic review of implementation and impacts. *PloS One,* 15(4), e0231350–e0231350. doi:10.1371/journal.pone.0231350

3

Improving health literacy in community settings

3.1 Introduction

In Chapter 2, we discussed health literacy tools and techniques that can be applied by health professionals working with patients and carers within a clinical environment. These methods tend to be more oriented to improving functional health literacy—achieving better patient understanding and compliance with recommended prevention, treatment and care. Despite the known advantages of shared decision-making, the practical constraints experienced in the clinical environment will often mean that the communication and educational methods we use do not facilitate a high level of interactive communication.

In this chapter, we examine a range of different community settings that provide opportunities for interventions that are more interactive. These interventions will often have specific behavioural goals but can be delivered in ways that also develop more generic health literacy skills that can be applied in different environments.

3.2 Health education and health literacy

Health education improves health literacy. Just as formally organised education is the main route to improved literacy in populations, it follows that organised and structured health education has the potential to improve health literacy. This can be limited to task-based communication—designed to develop specific skills to manage prescribed activities (medication adherence, behaviour change)—but can also be skills based—educational activities that are designed to develop more generic and transferable skills. These are skills that better equip people to discriminate between competing sources of information, adapt to changing circumstances and make more autonomous decisions relating to their health.

Health education has been an essential component of action to promote health and prevent disease for more than a century. Many campaigns have been and continue to be characterised by their emphasis on the transmission of information, often based upon a relatively simplistic understanding of the relationship between communication and behaviour change. This type of communication campaign may be helpful in improving essential health knowledge and can help improve functional health literacy. This is useful where discrete and relatively simple behavioural changes (such as immunisation uptake) are needed. However, these communications are generally much less successful in influencing more complex behaviour (such as food choices) and rarely achieve sustainable health behaviour change, especially when not accompanied by broader public health policy and regulations. Where health communication campaigns have been found to be effective, these successes have been most observable among the more economically advantaged in the community. They have made little impact on closing the gap in health status between different social and economic groups in society.

Health education has been considerably strengthened by the development of more sophisticated, theory-informed methods over recent decades. These theories are mainly drawn from social psychology and are not only focused on the transmission of information (though this remains important) but also the development of the personal and social skills that fit with contemporary concepts of interactive and critical health literacy. Consistent with the definition of health literacy in Chapter 1, these contemporary theories also incorporate the context of health decision-making, and enable people to develop the transferable personal and social skills that are required to make health-related decisions at different times and in different contexts across the life-course.

Several theories of behaviour change have helped to identify and explain the complex relationships between knowledge, beliefs and social context (see the References section and the companion volume to this book, *Theory in a Nutshell: a practical guide to health promotion theories*, for further information). These provide practical guidance on the content, sequencing and delivery of health education programs to improve interactive and critical health literacy, and support positive health-related decision-making in a variety of circumstances, emphasising:

- *Knowledge and beliefs about health:* improving individual knowledge about health and its determinants. Social cognitive theory, for example, highlights the importance of personalising health information, and of identifying health issues of most immediate relevance to people.
- *Self-efficacy:* an individual's belief in their capacity to act in the ways necessary to reach specific goals. The health belief model and social cognitive theory emphasise the importance of health education that helps people to develop confidence in their competence to make change. This can be achieved, for example, through personal observation, supervised practice and repetition. There is close alignment between improvement in self-efficacy and the development of more interactive and critical health literacy skills.

■ *Perceived social norms:* the value an individual places on social approval or acceptance by different social groups. Social cognitive theory and diffusion of innovation theory both highlight the influence of social role models, family and peer groups in supporting (or obstructing) change.

■ *Different stages of change:* stages of change theory describes how individuals in a population may be more or less receptive to health communications at different stages in their life. This understanding highlights the sequencing and targeting of health education messages to the right person at the right time across the life-course.

■ *Shaping or changing the environment* or people's perception of the environment: social cognitive theory highlights the important and continuing interactions between a person and their environment— reflecting the importance of interventions to reduce situational demands and complexity.

Testing and evaluation of health education interventions over several decades has highlighted the importance of the theoretical insights described in shaping more comprehensive and interactive forms of health communication. This approach to health communication is more obviously connected to the development of interactive and critical health literacy skills. It is through this focus on skills development and on empowerment that the concept of health literacy has, in turn, had a distinctive influence on the purpose and methodologies of health education and communication.

The following sections examine experience in improving health literacy among different settings and priority populations.

3.3   Health literacy interventions in different settings and across the life-course

Improving maternal health literacy

One of the classic "teachable moments" in the life-course is during pregnancy and early parenting. For first-time parents in particular, there is often high personal motivation to engage in health education, as well as opportunity and service accessibility. Although the data vary from country to country, around 50% of first-time parents attend formal antenatal education classes. These classes offer a unique opportunity to improve knowledge and develop skills to enable safe childbirth and successful parenting.

Past research has indicated that the methods and content of many of these programs is very limited. In content, the focus is often entirely on pregnancy and childbirth, missing an important opportunity to communicate and develop critical parenting skills and infant milestones. In method, the classes have traditionally been didactic and focused on the transmission of information rather than supporting interactive learning and the development of transferable health literacy skills.

Fortunately, this is changing and there are now some excellent examples of programs designed to improve maternal health literacy and systematically develop transferable skills for new parents. These are often built into existing points of connection between mothers and infants and healthcare providers rather than developed as "add-ons" to existing services. An example is provided in Case study 3.1.

CASE STUDY 3.1: The Parenting+ program

Researchers working closely with frontline health professionals and new parents in New South Wales (NSW), Australia, used the health literacy concept to develop a group-based training program for new parents. Known as Parenting+, the four-week program embeds health literacy skills into parenting topics of interest that have been identified by parents and family and child health nurses through consultation and piloting (see Figure 3.1).

Figure 3.1 Parenting Plus topics

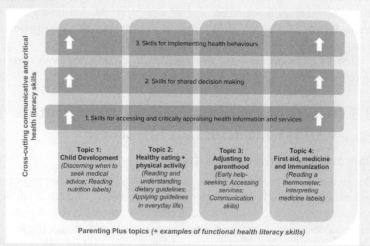

Parenting Plus topics (+ examples of functional health literacy skills)

Source: Muscat, D.M., Ayre, J., Harris, A., Tunchon, L., Zachariah, D., Nutbeam, D., & McCaffery, K. Using feasibility data and codesign to refine a group-based health literacy intervention for new parents. Health Literacy Research and Practice. 2021;5(4):e276-e282 https://doi.org/10.3928/24748307-20210911-01

(Continued)

Functional health literacy skills are specific to each content area in the Parenting+ program. These include skills to interpret medication dosage and timing instructions, measure temperature, understand nutritional labels and act on vaccination information, for example. To develop transferable health literacy skills applicable across contexts, three core skill sets are also included across all topics: (1) skills to access and critically appraise health information; (2) skills for shared decision-making; and (3) skills for implementing health behaviours.

The program makes use of already established baby health clinics and networks to develop with new parents the ability to "access, understand, appraise and use information" in ways that enable constructive interactions with healthcare providers, and support critical, independent application of new knowledge to promote and maintain their health and that of their children.

Health literacy interventions in schools

For obvious reasons, schools have long been identified as providing an ideal opportunity to help young people develop health knowledge and long-term, transferable health literacy skills. School health education has evolved from knowledge-based learning of essential facts and instruction on how to live, to far more sophisticated and comprehensive educational programs that are integrated into the overall learning experience of schools.

In considering the opportunity to improve the health literacy of school students, it is essential to keep in mind that the core business of schools is education, not health. Schools are assessed on their ability to optimise educational outcomes for students. Viewed within this context, schools should not be simply viewed as a convenient location for health topic-based interventions by those of us more focused on the achievement of improved health outcomes, such as to reduce tobacco or alcohol use, or promote healthy nutrition. Health education needs to contribute to the achievement of core education goals by addressing health issues within an education framework.

A focus on improving health literacy is helpful in reconciling the educational priority of schools and the health priorities that we may have. Schools provide a well-structured educational environment designed not only to develop students' knowledge, competencies and behaviours, but also their critical thinking and lifelong learning skills. This fits well with the concept of health literacy and offers a unique opportunity to work with students to develop interactive and critical health literacy skills.

This leads us to consider the more generic skills that can be achieved through school health literacy programs, rather than the instrumental, topic-based outcomes that have been characteristic of past school health education interventions. Broder and colleagues have provided a helpful review of potential outcomes from health literacy programs for children and adolescents that is useful in informing this reorientation. The authors concluded that health education in schools should occur over several years, be connected to young people's social and cognitive development, and be directed towards enabling children and adolescents to:

- better understand increasingly complex health information and discriminate between the high volume of information and educational materials accessible to them;
- become progressively responsible for their own health, for their use of health services and for dealing with different health-related issues;
- develop skills today that influence health (outcomes) and wellbeing over their life-course; and
- be able to construct their own views on health matters and communicate these to others.

This orientation towards the development of generic health literacy skills is not intended to be a complete substitution for more instrumental interventions to reduce tobacco, drug and alcohol use. Both can be achieved through carefully constructed contributions to the achievement of core education goals by addressing health issues within an education framework.

As with all school programs, past research into successful health interventions has also revealed consistent, practical requirements to achieve sustained change. These include educational materials for classroom use that are based on effective learning theories and tailored for the specific needs of young people at different stages in their social and cognitive development, and practical support for the professional development of teachers. Case study 3.2 The Informed Health Choices program exemplifies both the principle of embedding health within an educational framework and providing the practical tailored support referred to above.

CASE STUDY 3.2: The Informed Health Choices program

The Informed Health Choices program intervention was developed and tested in Uganda to help teach children aged 10- to 12-years how to assess claims about the benefits and harms of a range of actions intended to maintain or improve health. It covers key *interactive* and *critical* health literacy concepts helping students to develop skills in understanding and appraising health information. Informed Health Choices illustrates the way in which health literacy interventions can be developed for optimal delivery within the school setting:

- *Focus on generic skills rather than topic-based outcomes.* The goal of the Informed Health Choices program is to empower people not only to make better personal health choices but also to enable them to participate in community discussions as scientifically literate citizens by helping children to discriminate between different sources of health information and to construct and communicate their own views on health matters.
- *Provision of practical support.* The Informed Health Choices program includes a suite of learning resources for teachers and students, including a textbook, a teachers' guide, student exercise books, a poster and activity cards. Figure 3.2 provides an example from the textbook. Teachers were supported to implement the intervention through a 2-day workshop to familiarise themselves with the content and prepare a plan for delivering the lessons.
- *Focus on educational goals.* The intervention was implemented flexibly such that each participating school could decide how any usual academic content displaced by the Informed Health Choices lessons would be compensated. This helped to ensure that time was not taken away from other lessons and core educational business of each school.
- *Application of learning theory.* The Informed Health Choices intervention adopts a "spiral curriculum", introducing basic concepts first, repeating and reinforcing those in subsequent cycles, and introducing more difficult concepts later.

(Continued)

Figure 3.2 Informed Health Choices comic book

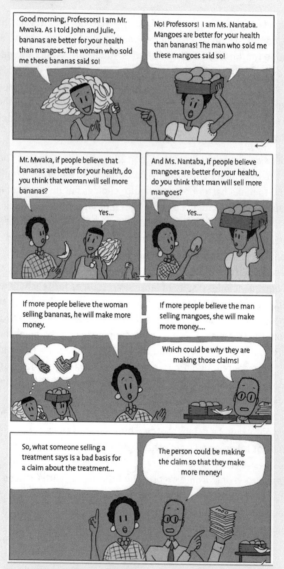

Source: Nsangi, A., Semakula, D., Oxman, A. D., Austvoll-Dahlgren, A., Oxman, M., et al., (2017). Effects of the Informed Health Choices primary school intervention on the ability of children in Uganda to assess the reliability of claims about treatment effects: a cluster-randomised controlled trial. The Lancet, 390(10092), 374-388. doi:10.1016/S0140-6736(17)31226-6

It is essential for those of us from health backgrounds to recognise the limitations of schools in solving complex health and social challenges created by powerful influences in families, communities and wider society. To optimise the contribution that schools make to health improvement and health literacy, the concept of a health promoting school has evolved as a way of linking health education in the school with wider family and community initiatives to promote health. The concept of a "health-literate school" fits within this wider framework and is discussed further in Chapter 5 on health-literate organisations.

There are several other school-based health literacy programs that have similarly been designed to ensure the best possible fit with the core educational goals of schools, and to provide health content guided by learning theory. In the US, for example, health literacy concepts have been built into lesson plans for second graders, including maths, language, arts, science and social studies (Aghazadeh et al. 2020). This approach addressed teacher concerns about the barriers of time, effort and new curriculum in a classroom's already packed schedule. Teachers, who were trained in health literacy and compensated for their time, generated trial sessions and lesson plans for use across a school district. Each lesson plan was required to meet at least one state standard in a core content area, such as reading or science, as well as one health literacy standard. Each lesson plan included an active learning component to increase comprehension of health literacy content and was able to be contextualised and tailored to students' daily lives and interests, helping to increase attention and learning. These examples from Uganda and the US show how health education informed by health literacy concepts can contribute to the achievement of schools' core education goals by addressing health issues within an education framework.

Adult education settings

In the same way that schools offer unmatched opportunities to help young people develop health literacy skills, partnerships between health and adult education organisations offer similar potential, especially in their access to socially disadvantaged groups. International literacy surveys have identified that a significant proportion of the adult population in most countries is assessed as illiterate/functionally illiterate. This ranges from up to 20% in the highest income countries, such as the US, UK and Australia, to 85%+ in some of the world's lowest income countries. These general literacy challenges are often caused or exacerbated by poor native language skills. This is most observable among migrants and refugees who may not have the native language of their adopted country as their first language.

Most countries have developed strategies and services to support the development of general language, literacy and numeracy (LLN) skills. These programs are often used by more socially and economically disadvantaged populations, specifically individuals with poor native language skills who may be participating in English as a second language (ESL) programs. Opportunities exist to partner with adult literacy providers to integrate health content into adult education programs. As students develop their basic language, literacy and numeracy skills, integrating health content into the curriculum concurrently can help students develop their health literacy skills.

There are now some excellent working examples of partnerships between health practitioners and organisations and adult LLN programs that have successfully integrated health content into adult learning. Where evaluations have been conducted, they have shown that:

- all forms of adult LLN programs will help improve health literacy (regardless of whether health is incorporated into the curriculum content);
- programs that incorporate health content provide added value by improving specific health knowledge as well as more advanced health literacy skills alongside improvements in general LLN skills;
- both teachers and participants in programs with health content place value on the specific content and connection to the "real world"; and
- participation, engagement and continuing attendance rates are enhanced by inclusion of health content.

Growing practical experience indicates several steps that are common in building such partnerships. Similar to schools, effective partnerships begin with respect for the core business of adult education organisations in developing generic language, literacy and numeracy skills. Our goal is to add mutually beneficial value within this context. The added value we bring as health practitioners is in our content knowledge and ability to mobilise resources to support greater health content in adult LLN programs. Exactly as with schools, past experience indicates that successful adoption requires educational materials for classroom use that are based on effective learning theories and tailored for the specific needs of adult learners, and practical support for the professional development of teachers.

There now exist several working examples of curriculum content of proven efficacy that can be delivered by non-health professionals to adult learners. For example, a systematic review of ESL health literacy curriculum identified several distinct curricula (Chen et al., 2015). Each helped students to develop functional health literacy, with a majority incorporating higher level (interactive and critical) health literacy skills. A smaller number of curricula addressed critical health literacy through the inclusion of elements of social justice and empowerment, including health advocacy in the community. Overall, evaluations indicated that all were effective in improving

ESL students' English reading scores (core business) *and* health literacy as assessed by validated measures and/or knowledge related to specific health conditions. A clear win–win.

In terms of professional development, experience from successful programs indicates that this is essential but not necessarily onerous for either partner. For example, in Case study 3.3 from Australia, in response to differentiated requests from the teachers, health professionals provided support that ranged from four hours to six half-day sessions to familiarise the adult education teachers with the health content of the curriculum.

Taken as a whole, these practical experiences provide compelling evidence for health practitioner and health organisation partnerships with adult education organisations to improve health literacy in disadvantaged populations.

CASE STUDY 3.3: The "Living Literacy" Health Literacy program

A health skills education program based on the UK *Skilled for Health* program was adapted for delivery through established adult basic education classes in NSW, Australia. It had dual aims of improving participants' health literacy as well as their core LLN skills as prescribed by the Australian Core Skills Framework. Key LLN skills were embedded within materials containing health-related topics focused on public health priorities. Students learnt specified LLN skills through engaging with health material guided by their teacher. Topics included functional (e.g. taking temperatures; checking medicine labels) through to communicative (e.g. answering your doctor's questions) and critical health literacy (e.g. shared decision-making) skills.

Adult education teachers were supported to deliver health content by two teaching manuals and a suggested delivery plan which could be applied flexibly, according to the interests and capabilities of students. The main requirement for delivery was that classes cover all 10 "core" topics considered central to the health literacy learning objectives. Through the partnership, adult education centres derived additional benefit through connection with local community health services and health professionals. Instructions for the collaboration were not prescriptive to permit flexibility. Health professionals spent variable time in providing support, ranging from four hours to six half-days engaging with the program (including preparation, class visit and follow-up).

Evaluations of the Living Literacy program showed that both the standard LLN program and health literacy program benefited

(Continued)

participants, with improvements in functional health literacy (e.g. reading a thermometer), confidence in health decision-making and other health literacy domains. Students in the health literacy program had better outcomes with more advanced health literacy skills, greater confidence and higher health knowledge scores after six months. The health professionals who participated felt this project was a good fit for their role and valued the partnership with adult educators. The adult educators provided positive feedback on the feasibility of teaching and receptivity of students. (McCaffery et al.,2019)

Community health literacy programs for older adults

As people age, their health needs become more complex and health services use more frequent. Numerous studies have identified that inadequate health literacy is more common among older adults than the rest of the population. Considerable attention has been given to the impact of poor health literacy among older adults on their health services use, chronic disease management and health outcomes. Many of the methodologies described in Chapter 2 have been applied with success among older adults in hospital, clinic and community health settings.

First diagnosis with a chronic disease, such as diabetes, often provides a "teachable moment" described earlier. Health and civil society organisations have developed patient education materials and programs to respond optimally to these challenges and opportunities, mostly focused on improving functional health literacy in ways that enable patients to contribute successfully to disease self-management. Some of these programs reflect a more sophisticated understanding of health education and communication described in this chapter, but many others are not oriented to the needs of patients with lower health literacy skills and can be improved through the application of more sophisticated educational methods.

Separate to these important and necessary interventions in healthcare, increasing attention has been given to community-based programs to improve interactive and critical health literacy among older adults in the community. These interventions have a variety of goals: to improve disease prevention; to enable people to find trustworthy and relevant health information; and to support improved understanding of the determinants of health and encourage actions to change those influences.

Critical themes for successfully working with older community members have emerged from research and practical experience. First among these is the issue of "trust" and, related to this, the quality of relationships between learners and between educator and learner (Brooks et al., 2017). This is a consistent theme at all life stages but especially important with older adults.

A recommended approach to building trust is through collaborative learning, or co-learning. Co-learning usually involves creating a learning environment where older adults can interact and exchange health knowledge and experiences with family, community members or peers alongside healthcare professionals in order to learn from each other. Case study 3.4 from Brazil provides an example of this.

Research has also shown that social support is important in developing more advanced interactive and critical health literacy skills in older adults. Social support may be emotional (by sharing experiences), instrumental (by providing practical assistance), informational (by providing advice and information) and as critical friend (information for self-evaluation). These types of social support can contribute to people's understanding and ability to judge, sift and use health information. A commitment to collaborative learning—creating a learning environment in which participants can safely interact and exchange health knowledge peer to peer—can also facilitate mutually beneficial social support.

CASE STUDY 3.4: The Alfa-Health program

The Alfa-Health program is an educational program designed to improve critical health literacy among older adults in Brazil. The focus was on developing transferable skills that equip people to make a range of more autonomous decisions relating to their health, and to adapt to changing circumstances. The intervention was conducted by a nurse over a 20-week period through weekly meetings in a group room in the public healthcare unit. The main topics focused on access to the health system, safe use of medicines, healthy lifestyle choices, the use of prevention services, mental health, men's and women's health, human rights, social participation, retirement and healthy environments.

In interviews, participants consistently identified the benefits of social support from belonging to the Alfa-Health group. For many, this was expressed in a context in which they previously rarely left their homes or had wanted to. Such reflections situated the program as a beneficial yet unique space where older adults could come together. Social cohesion within the group appeared to be facilitated by classroom practices which enabled the sharing of health information and respect for personal experience. Older adults found commonalities in shared health experiences and challenges, which brought the group together and this was perceived to have facilitated learning.

The program helped older adults living in a highly disadvantaged community to gain skills and confidence in their health decision-making, to engage successfully with health professionals and to navigate the healthcare system (Serbim et al.,2020).

Distributed health literacy

As a final consideration in this chapter, almost all of the examples discussed focus on developing individual health literacy skills. This reflects the ways in which health literacy is generally conceptualised, measured and improved through intervention in defined populations and communities. However, this individual orientation doesn't fully reflect the lived experience of many of us in our families and communities. For many of us, our individual health literacy skills are supplemented by those of others we have access to (including our family, carers, work colleagues and health professionals). Such collective knowledge and skills have been described as "distributed health literacy" and defined as "the health literacy abilities, skills and practices of others that contribute to an individual's level of health literacy" (Edwards et al., 2015). This conceptualisation of health literacy recognises that a group of individuals may each possess only limited health literacy skills, but by combining their knowledge and skills can achieve mutual, collective benefit through improved health literacy.

Early research into this concept has illustrated how health literacy is "distributed" through family and social networks, and that it is common for people to draw on the health literacy skills of others to seek, understand and use health information. Those who passed on their health literacy skills act as health literacy mediators and supported others in accessing and understanding specific health information. Access to this wider network of information, skills and experience enabled people to better manage their health, become more active in healthcare decision-making processes and more effectively communicate with health professionals.

Thinking about health literacy in this way is a reminder of the ways in which a person's social network can influence their health literacy through shared health knowledge, supported skills and practices, and health-related decisions. In this way, community-based health literacy interventions have the potential to have distributed impacts—through family, school, workplace and wider community "ripple effects". The practical implication of the concept is that it reinforces the importance of enabling social networks and social support as an important part of health literacy interventions for adults and reminds us to actively consider the potential ripple effects of interventions we are organising within a community setting.

It is also the case that health misinformation can emerge from social networks and that these ripple effects can have a negative impact on health literacy as well as a positive impact. This is an issue we examine more closely in Chapter 4 Digital health literacy.

3.4 Summary

Health education improves health literacy: Health education remains a fundamental intervention for improving public health in communities. Decades of research and practical experience have identified communication methodologies that are not only effective in improving knowledge, but also in developing transferable health literacy skills. These methodologies highlight the need to tailor communications to the different needs of individuals and communities, to incorporate people's perceptions of social context and social norms, and to support people in building confidence in their decision-making (self-efficacy).

Interactive communication builds skills and confidence: Differences in communication methods, media and content will result in different learning outcomes. Developing transferable skills, supporting critical thinking about the determinants of health and empowering people to act require a substantially different approach to health communication in both methods and content. It prompts the use of more interactive and adaptable communication methods (to incorporate personal preferences and enable development of skills) and a widening of content in many instances. Through this focus on skills development and empowerment, health literacy has a distinctive influence on the purpose and methodologies of traditional health education and communication.

Key principles for effective community programs: There are several community settings that provide unique opportunities to develop health literacy through partnerships across the life-course. Though each is different in the access it provides to different populations, there are some important common features that help optimise the potential to improve health literacy. These include:

■ **Respect for the core business of partners,** especially in educational settings—recognising the need to address health issues within an educational framework.

■ **Development of educational materials** that are practical for use, interactive for students/learners and support the development of enduring health literacy skills.

■ **Training support for educators** who may be unfamiliar with the communication methods and health content they are being asked to work with.

■ **Collaborative learning** to create trust and mutual respect between learners and between educator and learner, especially by engaging adult learners in the development of health education materials and methods.

■ **Mobilising social support and networks** by creating a learning environment in which participants can safely interact and exchange health knowledge.

References

Aghazadeh SA, Aldoory L, Mills T 2020. Integrating health literacy into core curriculum: a teacher-driven pilot initiative for second graders. *Journal of School Health,* 90, 585–593. doi:10.1111/josh.12907

Bröder J, Okan O, Bauer U, Bruland D, Schlupp S, et al. 2017. Health literacy in childhood and youth: a systematic review of definitions and models. *BMC Public Health,* 17(1), 361–361. doi:10.1186/s12889-017-4267-y

Brooks C, Ballinger C, Nutbeam D, Adams J 2017. The importance of building trust and tailoring interactions when meeting older adults' health literacy needs. *Disability and Rehabilitation,* 39(23), 2428–2435. doi:10.1080/09638288.2016.1231849

Chen X, Goodson P, Acosta S 2015. Blending health literacy with an english as a second language curriculum: a systematic literature review. *Journal of Health Communication,* 20(2), 101–111. doi:10.1080/10810730.2015.1066467

Edwards M, Wood F, Davies M, Edwards A 2015. "Distributed health literacy": longitudinal qualitative analysis of the roles of health literacy mediators and social networks of people living with a long-term health condition. *Health Expectations,* 18(5), 1180–1193. doi:10.1111/hex.12093

McCaffery KJ, Morony S, Muscat DM, Hayen A, Shepherd HL, et al. 2019. Evaluation of an Australian health literacy program delivered in adult education settings. *Health Literacy Research and Practice,* 3(3), S42–57. doi:10.3928/24748307-20190402-01

Muscat DM, Ayre J, Harris A, Tunchon L, Zachariah D, et al. 2021. Using feasibility data and codesign to refine a group-based health literacy intervention for new parents. *Health Literacy Research and Practice,* 5(4), e276-e282. doi:10.3928/24748307-20210911-01

Nsangi A, Semakula D, Oxman AD, Austvoll-Dahlgren A, Oxman M, et al. 2017. Effects of the Informed Health Choices primary school intervention on the ability of children in Uganda to assess the reliability of claims about treatment effects: a cluster-randomised controlled trial. *Lancet,* 390(10092), 374–388. doi:10.1016/S0140-6736(17)31226-6

Serbim A, Paskulin L, Nutbeam D 2020. Improving health literacy among older people through primary health care units in Brazil: feasibility study. *Health Promotion International,* 35(6), 1256–1266. doi:10.1093/heapro/daz121

Further reading

Blennow M, Ekroth Porcel M, Fassih N, Frenzel L, Heimer Å, et al. 2013. Annual report on child health, 2012. Stockholm, Sweden: Department of Child Health Services, Stockholm County Council. Retrieved from: http://www.webbhotell.sll.se/Global/Bhv/Dokument/Rapporter/

Lawson PJ, Flocke SA 2009. Teachable moments for health behavior change: a concept analysis. *Patient Education and Counseling,* 76(1), 25–30. doi:10.1016/j.pec.2008.11.002

Nutbeam D, Harris E, Wise M 2022. *Theory in a Nutshell: a practical guide to health promotion theories* (4th edition). Sydney, McGraw Hill Education Australia Pty Ltd.

Paakkari L, Paakkari O 2012. Health literacy as a learning outcome in schools. *Health Education,* 112(2), 133–152. doi:10.1108/09654281211203411

St Leger L 2001. Schools, health literacy and public health: possibilities and challenges. *Health Promotion International,* 16(2), 197–205. doi:10.1093/heapro/16.2.197

4

Digital health literacy

4.1 Introduction

When looking for information and advice on most issues, the vast majority of people will now turn to digital sources of information as a starting point. Historically, access to relevant, timely information has been a major obstacle for many. Today, access is no longer an issue for most people as they obtain information from a vast array of online sources, including internet websites, mobile applications (apps) and social media. Search engines such as Google have streamlined the process of finding health information. The application of evolving artificial intelligence (AI) technologies is increasing options for searching as well as organising search results in ever more sophisticated forms. The problem is much less one of access, but rather of finding relevant, trustworthy and usable information in a largely unregulated landscape. This is as true for people looking for health information and advice as it is for any other form of information.

To match the growth in access and use of digital media by the public, use of digital media for health communication has also grown exponentially over the past 20 years. Communication providers—the government, health and civil society organisations, as well as private for-profit organisations—have invested heavily in the development of websites and apps for digital devices, as well as engaging with social media to get their messages to different target populations.

Digital technology has brought us many new tools for health promotion, addressing a wide range of access and cost challenges that have been limitations to health education programs in the past. These technologies enable us to communicate directly with large numbers of people at relatively low cost. They offer unprecedented opportunities to target and personalise information and to engage people in interactive communication.

The great opportunity of digital technology has also created new challenges. It has not only made it easier to access valuable health information, but also provided equally easy access to information and opinion that is inaccurate, sometimes deliberately misleading and often driven by commercial motive. The marketplace for health communication is more crowded and complex than at any time before.

For those of us who want to get our health messages in the right form, to the right person at the right time, the opportunities are great but the competition for attention even greater. This requires us to consider very carefully the quality of messaging and optimal use of different media. For those searching for health information, such a crowded marketplace has required the development of a range of new literacy skills, especially those required to assess the usefulness of different digital media, as well as relevance and trustworthiness of the many and varied sources of health information. These skills are referred to as *eHealth literacy,* and increasingly commonly as *digital health literacy.*

In this chapter, we examine the concept of eHealth literacy and focus attention on the ways in which we can develop and optimise online resources that ensure we get the right message in the right form to the right person. Well-designed resources can also help overcome the challenge of lower health literacy, as well as help people to develop eHealth literacy skills and avoid the proliferation of misinformation and disinformation that is accessible online.

4.2 What is eHealth literacy?

eHealth literacy is generally defined as "the ability to seek, find, understand, and appraise health information from digital sources and apply the knowledge gained to addressing or solving a health problem" (Norman & Skinner, 2006). As is the case with generic health literacy skills, eHealth literacy skills are influenced by an individual's general literacy, numeracy and educational background, the context in which they are seeking health information (their health status and medical experience), motivation for seeking the information, as well as experience with the technologies used.

The concept of eHealth literacy has evolved. Norgaard and colleagues have developed a comprehensive eHealth Literacy Framework (eHLF), illustrated in Figure 4.1. This model distinguishes between:

- the attributes of users (1–2: knowledge about their health; ability to process information);
- the interaction between users and the technologies (3–5: ability to actively engage with digital technologies; their feeling of being safe and in control; and their motivation for using digital technologies); and
- users' experience of systems (6–7: the technology works, is accessible and suits users' needs).

The model also distinguishes between the influence of more externalised, visible actions (such as observing others) to more internalised concepts and feelings (self-efficacy) on the vertical axis.

Figure 4.1 Framework for eHealth literacy

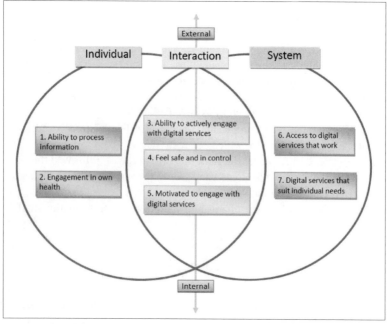

Source: Norgaard, O., Furstrand, D., Klokker, L., Karnoe, A., Batterham, R., Kayser, L., & Osborne, R. H. (2015). The e-health literacy framework: A conceptual framework for characterizing e-health users and their interaction with e-health systems. Knowledge Management & e-Learning, 7(4), 522–540. doi:10.34105/j.kmel.2015.07.035

The importance of this model is that it not only focuses our attention on the attributes of individuals and on the technology (its ease of access and usefulness), but also on the interaction between the two. The model emphasises the balance of individual attributes and skills and the complexity of the system/environment in which they are to be used in a very similar way to the general model for health literacy in Chapter 1.

Improving eHealth literacy requires us to focus at least as much on the ways we can reduce the complexity of the information system and environment as it does on helping people develop specific skills to enable them to identify and engage productively with relevant, trustworthy sources of information on digital platforms. The following sections focus on ways we can create websites, apps and other digital communications in ways that are more accessible to individuals with lower health literacy and eHealth literacy. This includes design features that invite people to find relevant and trustworthy information, support interactive learning and help those accessing digital information to develop interactive and critical health literacy skills.

4.3   Developing digital tools for health literacy

There are now hundreds of thousands of websites and apps for digital devices that provide health information, advice and opinion. Reviews of the usefulness of different websites and apps (listed at the end of the Chapter) have demonstrated their great potential to reach different populations in low-, middle- and high-income countries, and to be useful aids to health decision-making. Disappointingly, research has also shown, time and again, that online health information is provided on websites that are poorly designed and hard to navigate, greatly reducing accessibility and utility. Health websites frequently use language at a level that is too difficult for most people to read and understand. Too few take full advantage of the opportunities offered by digital platforms; for example, to create interactive and personalised features, and to provide feedback to those using the sites. All consumers seeking health information online face challenges in easily identifying reliable and trustworthy sources of information that are free from commercial influences.

While many of us engaged in health education and patient education have embraced the great potential of digital technologies, too often we fail to fully capitalise on that potential and, in doing so, may also exacerbate existing inequities in health associated with poorer literacy and language skills. The onus is on us to get it right and there are excellent resources to help in doing so. This section provides guidance on tools and methods for optimising the reliability, utility and impact of digital communications.

Information reliability

Information reliability refers to the accuracy and credibility of online content, as well as transparency in the purpose and ownership of the site. This information is essential in enabling users to better understand both the origin and quality of online content. In practice, it means that it should be easy for users to quickly identify the source of the information (government, civil society, commercial) and more easily understand its purposes. Reporting on the underlying source of advice (evidence) and the timing of the most recent update of that information is also helpful in building consumer confidence in the reliability of the information.

In Table 4.1, Devine and colleagues (2016) provide a helpful summary of some of the most important requirements and features of websites that can be used to improve consumer perceptions of their reliability. This type of checklist provides a helpful prompt for those of us involved in designing and updating health websites. It can also help us in our work with consumers and patients in identifying reliable sources of health information by highlighting key features of trustworthy websites.

Table 4.1 Making quality health websites: Reliability requirements

Criteria	Reliability requirements
Identity	1. Name of person or organisation responsible for website
	2. Street address for person or organisation responsible for website
	3. Identified source of funding for website
Purpose	4. Statement of purpose or mission for website
	5. Uses and limitations of services provided
	6. Association with commercial products or services
Content development	7. Differentiation of advertising from non-advertising content
	8. Medical, editorial, or quality review practices or policies
	9. Authorship of health content (per page of health content)
Privacy	10. Privacy policy
	11. How personal information is protected
User feedback	12. Feedback form or mechanism
	13. How information from users is used
Content updating	14. Date content created (per page of health content)
	15. Date content reviewed, updated, modified or revised (per page of health content)
	16. Copyright date

Source: Devine T, Broderick J, Harris LM, Wu H, Hilfiker SW 2016. Making quality health websites a national public health priority: toward quality standards. Journal of Medical Internet Research, 18(8), e211. doi:10.2196/jmir.5999.

Website usability

Website usability is commonly considered in three major categories. The first focuses on how the information is organised, often referred to as "information architecture". The second concerns how users navigate the information on a website, often referred to as "site design". The third focuses on how users interact with content on the website, referred to as "content design". Usability is a fundamental element of assessing website quality, having a profound impact on ease of access to the information a consumer is looking for, and their ability to understand and personalise information. The time (and resources) invested in making a website easy to use are generally

Table 4.2 Making quality health websites: Usability requirements

Categories	Established usability principles
Site design	1. Use conventional interaction elements
	2. Make it obvious what is clickable and what is not
	3. Minimise vertical scrolling
	4. Ensure that the Back button behaves predictably
	5. Provide clear feedback signals for actions
	6. Ensure site is accessible for users with disabilities
	7. Provide a simplified user experience
	8. Incorporate multimedia
	9. Offer a functional home page
Information architecture	10. Present a clear visual hierarchy
	11. Provide easy search functionality
	12. Clearly label content categories
	13. Make pages easy to skim or scan
	14. Make elements on the page easy to read
	15. Visually group related topics
	16. Make sure text and background colors contrast
Content design	17. Focus the writing on audience and purpose
	18. Use the users' language; minimise jargon and technical terms
	19. Allow for interaction with the content

Source: Devine T, Broderick J, Harris LM, Wu H, Hilfiker SW 2016. Making quality health websites a national public health priority: toward quality standards. Journal of Medical Internet Research, 18(8), e211. doi:10.2196/jmir.5999.

critical in its successful use. The standards for success are high. We are often competing for consumer attention with high-quality commercial websites. People's tolerance for poorly designed websites is low.

In Table 4.2, Devine and colleagues (2016) again provide a useful tabular summary of some of the key issues that need to be considered in ensuring optimal "usability" for the website and app users. This checklist similarly provides a helpful prompt for those designing and updating health websites and can help us in our work with consumers and patients in highlighting key features of the most useful websites.

Website engagement

In Chapter 2, we introduced common methods for simplifying written health information, including through readability testing and the application of tools such as the Patient Education Materials Assessment Tool (PEMAT). While these methods can and should be applied to the development of online health information, there are some additional considerations for presenting information in online formats. These focus not only on the importance of using simplified language but also on a range of presentational issues that make best use of the opportunities of online screen presentations and minimise the limitations.

The US Office of Disease Prevention and Health Promotion (ODPHP) has developed *Health Literacy Online,* a research-based guide to help people develop intuitive health websites and digital tools that can be easily accessed and understood by all users. The guide contains a range of strategies with examples for writing and designing health websites that are accessible to users with limited literacy skills.

In addition to the generic advice to simplify language, *Health Literacy Online* provides clear advice on the need to develop "actionable" content. It reminds us that web users want to quickly and easily understand the health issue that has brought them to the website and find out how to take action—what they can do to address the problem. Content needs to be brief and to the point, engaging and actionable—informing users what you want them to do and providing practical steps to do it.

The guidance reminds us that there is good evidence to show that high levels of engagement with online health information are most likely to lead to health behaviour change and recommends the use of a range of interactive tools and strategies. Using multimedia like video, audio and graphics are effective ways to engage users. For consumers, this might include options to watch video testimonials of people like them or quizzes, buttons and links to other (reliable) sources of information. It's also important to make it convenient for users to share content with their online networks by adding social media buttons to your website.

Finally, it is important to remember that in developing an engaging website or app, writing simplified content that is easy-to-read is only part of the challenge in preparing online resources. Even health content written in plain language can look overwhelming if there's too much text in a paragraph or not enough "white space" on the page in view. The content layout, font and colour can help users understand the content on your website.

Optimising the use of mobile devices

Almost all the advice in the preceding section was originally developed to support the creation and improvement of websites. Today, many (if not a majority of people) access websites on mobile devices. Over time, this advice has been adapted and updated to apply to website use on mobile devices and progressively for use in the development of mobile apps.

There has been phenomenal growth in the number of health-related apps available to download to mobile devices. These offer many new possibilities to make health communication more attractive and effective. Apps have been developed to enable health information to be tailored to specific user needs or preferences; provide convenient, real-time access to features that collect and visualise personal data; and provide real-time feedback, set goals and provide prompts for future action. These apps can engage consumers in ways that help develop the knowledge, skills and confidence that reflect more interactive and critical health literacy skills. Case study 4.1 provides an example of ways in which the interactive features of an app can be used to help develop health literacy skills.

Commercial organisations have been the biggest drivers of the growth in health-related app development, often associated with other commercially valuable digital technology such as wearable devices. Relatively few of the commercially developed apps have been subjected to meaningful evaluation and (as is the case generally with the use of the internet and digital devices) their uptake has generally been strongest among younger, wealthier and better educated populations. This is a reminder that there remains a "digital divide" in access to and use of digital media that has potential to exacerbate existing inequities in health. As is always the case in considering communication media and messaging, it is essential to take account of patterns of access and use of digital media in the populations you are working with (Sieck et al., 2021).

Many health organisations have also recognised the potential of health apps and there is growing experience with their use across the full spectrum of health promotion through to disease management. Results from evaluations of these apps are variable but demonstrate some potential, often as an extension to other forms of communication and professional support. Reviews of the usefulness of health apps indicate that most have not been developed with the needs and preferences of people with lower health literacy skills in mind, strongly reinforcing the importance of systematically engaging target populations in the development of apps (and all forms of digital communication).

CASE STUDY 4.1: The SUCCESS app

The SUCCESS app is an Australian app developed for adults living with chronic kidney disease, searchable on the App Store and Google Play (Muscat et al., 2021). The app was designed to include tailored information for people receiving dialysis. It was developed using strategies to (a) reduce textual complexity, as well as features to (b) improve the communicative and critical health literacy skills of patients. In regards to the former, this included:

- lowering grade reading scores
- improving understandability and actionability using the Patient Education Materials Assessment Tool (PEMAT)
- incorporating video demonstrations, text-to-speech functions, micro-learning tasks and interactive quizzes.

To build patient skills, SUCCESS included:

- *Question prompt lists* to help patients to identify questions they wish to ask their healthcare team
- *Volitional help sheets* to plan for behavioural changes (e.g. planning to have less fluids)
- *Animated training* in:
  - healthcare communication
  - shared decision-making
  - critical appraisal of online information.

In this way, the app was designed to be both engaging and actionable, informing users what to do, providing practical steps, and helping develop the skills and confidence to take those steps. The inclusion of skills training related to the critical appraisal of online information also served as a way to tackle misinformation and disinformation, which is discussed further below in this chapter.

4.4   Tackling misinformation and disinformation

The promise of digital communication can be severely compromised by reliability of online information. The same digital technologies that make it easier to access quality health information have also provided easy access to information and opinion that is inaccurate and sometimes deliberately misleading. This challenge has been acutely observable throughout the COVID-19 pandemic, amplified by the widespread availability of misinformation and disinformation about the causes, management and consequences of COVID-19—especially through social media. This made it difficult for many to access, understand and act on reliable, trustworthy information at the time they needed it most.

As the extent of COVID-19 misinformation and disinformation became clear, the Director General of the World Health Organization (WHO) described the phenomenon as an "infodemic". It required governments and health organisations (including and especially the WHO) to respond to the public need for reliable, trustworthy information, as well as action to address the misinformation and myths that had the capacity to derail broader public health actions to control the pandemic.

While the COVID-19 pandemic brought this issue to public attention, the extent and range of inaccurate and misleading health information ranges far wider to include vaccines, especially human papilloma virus; illegal drugs and tobacco use; non-communicable diseases, especially cancer; eating disorders; and medical treatments. This is most pronounced among social media.

Past research has indicated that a majority of people use low-quality websites when looking for health information, including those with higher levels of health literacy. Participants in one study were asked to search for answers to six common health questions and were then monitored as to whether they used accredited sites or unaccredited sites such as blogs. Ninety-six per cent of individuals used an unaccredited source for at least one question (Quinn et al., 2017). Even when consumers are able to distinguish between trustworthy and untrustworthy sites, they may not engage with high-quality information if the low-quality information is easier to understand and/ or more interactive.

This and other research provide a compelling reminder for those of us creating online content of the need to make sure that our educational content is easy to understand and engaging for consumers. It needs to "compete" with many alternative sources of information on the quality of presentation.

In keeping with the approaches to improving health literacy described in Chapter 1, responding to inaccurate and deliberately misleading information online requires complementary strategies to improve both the accessibility of quality online information and support for people in effectively navigating to trustworthy sources of information.

During the COVID-19 pandemic, the WHO developed a number of useful tools for governments and health organisations, as well as information and resources that were intended for use directly by the general public to combat misinformation. These included a competency framework for health authorities and institutions to manage infodemics and a "Mythbusters" infographic series. These provide good models for an effective response to inaccurate and misleading information online. Links to these websites and other useful resources are provided at the end of the chapter.

4.5   Developing eHealth literacy skills

The COVID-19 "infodemic" provided a sharp reminder of the importance of managing the information environment while concurrently helping people develop their health literacy skills. As governments around the world struggle to find the best way to regulate the quality of online information and the platforms that distribute that information, much of the responsibility for finding reliable, accurate health information online rests with the consumer and those of us working directly with consumers.

Like other literacies, eHealth literacy is not static. It can be developed through personal experience and more deliberate exposure to educational structures and processes that support interactive learning and skills development. As with general health literacy, improving eHealth literacy involves developing the skills and confidence that empower individuals and enable them to fully participate in health decisions informed by successful engagement with digital technologies. These skills are not fixed for all time and require continued learning and adaptation across the life-course. Digital technologies continue to develop; for example, the rapid evolution of AI and its influence on a growing range of consumer activities. As these technologies change, so too must the concept of eHealth literacy.

There are a growing number of examples of programs designed to strengthen consumer eHealth literacy. As with more general health literacy programs discussed in Chapter 3, these have often been directed at "teachable moments" in the life-course, such as parenting, at school age children and at older adults. These have shown that it is possible to develop practical skills in identifying and using trustworthy health information websites, especially when interventions are linked to the health communication concepts and theories described in Chapter 2. Case study 4.2 describes an example of this type of intervention with parents of children with complex medical conditions.

There are also some practical tools and models that are becoming more commonly used, often embedded within existing patient and community health education programs. One example of this is the Trust It or Trash It model for appraisal of the quality of health information. This model encourages consumers to consider three questions in appraising whether or not a website should be trusted:

- *Who said it?*—encouraging consumers to critically consider who wrote it, where did the facts come from and who paid for it;
- *When did they say it?*—making sure that the information is current; and
- *How did they know?*—encouraging consumers to critically consider whether the information is based on the work of many people and seems reasonable on the basis of what they know.

This offers a simple, practical methodology to support patients and consumers in engaging critically with online information and provides clear advice on websites that can be trusted, and those that are best ignored. This type of checklist can be easily incorporated into a range of in-person and online educational programs.

CASE STUDY 4.2: The Good Googling program

The Good Googling program was developed for parents of children with complex medical conditions. The main objectives of the program were to "teach parents how and where to look for reliable health information online, how to form a searchable question, how to share their findings with their healthcare providers and how to use information delivery shortcuts such as email alerts. In this way, the program promoted interactive and critical eHealth literacy skills" (Armstrong-Heimsoth et al., 2017, p. 116).

Specifically, participants were taught to critically appraise website quality by examining specific features (e.g. currency, authorship, website domain) and by applying tools (e.g. the Trust It or Trash It tool [mentioned in the text earlier]). Participants were also taught how to search research databases, determine the quality of research and access further information as needed. They were then shown how to record the findings of their research and share them with their healthcare providers using purpose-designed communication sheets.

The Good Googling program included 60 minutes of face-to-face instruction and was delivered by an occupational therapist (OT) and

(Continued)

four OT doctoral students, with support from a university librarian and a representative from a paediatric consumer health library. Evaluation of the program found significant improvements in confidence related to: finding quality health information online, judging trustworthiness of online health information, understanding health information and using email alerts to retrieve information.

While the Good Googling program included a number of high-level eHealth literacy skills, other programs focus on less complex and more functional skills. Programs for older adults, for example, have included skills to support seniors in their navigation of specific government health websites or on how to be safe while searching for health information on the internet.

4.6 Summary

Digital technologies require digital health literacy: Digital technologies enable us to communicate directly with large numbers of people at relatively low cost as well as offering opportunities to target and personalise information and to engage people in interactive communication. Those searching for health information online require *eHealth literacy* skills to *seek, find, understand and appraise health information from digital sources.* Improving eHealth literacy requires us to focus substantially on the ways we can reduce the complexity of the information system and environment alongside helping people develop eHealth literacy skills.

Getting the right message in the right form to the right person: The competition for attention across multiple platforms for digital communication is great. Those of us creating online content need to make sure that our content is easy to understand and engaging for consumers. The onus is on us as information providers to ensure we get the right message in the right form to the right person. Online health information delivered through websites, mobile apps or social media needs to be relevant, trustworthy, accessible and engaging in ways that support action. There are several practical steps that need to be taken to ensure that this is delivered to consumers. These include:

- **Trust:** Information and features that build trust in the quality, relevance and timeliness of the content.

- **Access:** Platform and message features that make information accessible, understandable and navigable.
- **Engagement:** Optimal use of the technology to support interactive learning, message personalisation, feedback and monitoring.

Improving digital health literacy: Like other literacies, eHealth literacy is not static. It can be developed through personal experience and exposure to educational structures and processes that support people to optimally *seek, find, understand and appraise health information from digital sources.* There are some emerging examples of tools, programs and program content that is focused on improving eHealth literacy in specific populations, most notably directed at school students and older adults. These help patients and consumers to:

- **Discriminate**—across sources of information to identify trustworthy online information;
- **Navigate**—the platform to make best use of the available technology to engage in interactive learning; and
- **Critique**—content, messaging and purpose.

As with general health literacy, improving eHealth literacy involves developing the skills and confidence that enable people to fully participate in health decisions informed by successful engagement with digital technologies.

References

Armstrong-Heimsoth A, Johnson ML, McCulley A, Basinger M, Maki K, et al. 2017. Good Googling: a consumer health literacy program empowering parents to find quality health information online. *Journal of Consumer Health on the Internet*, 21(2), 111–124. doi:10.1080/15398285.2017.1308191

Devine T, Broderick J, Harris LM, Wu H, Hilfiker SW 2016. Making quality health websites a national public health priority: toward quality standards. *Journal of Medical Internet Research*, 18(8), e211. doi:10.2196/jmir.5999

Muscat DM, Lambert K, Shepherd H, McCaffery KJ, Zwi S, et al. 2021. Supporting patients to be involved in decisions about their health and care: development of a best practice health literacy App for Australian adults living with Chronic Kidney Disease. *Health Promotion Journal of Australia*, 32, 115–127. doi:10.1002/hpja.416

Norgaard O, Furstrand D, Klokker L, Karnoe A, Batterham R, et al. 2015. The e-health literacy framework: a conceptual framework for characterizing e-health users and their interaction with e-health systems. *Knowledge Management & E-Learning*, 7(4), 522–540. doi:10.34105/j.kmel.2015.07.035

Norman C, Skinner H 2006. eHealth literacy: essential skills for consumer health in a networked world. *Journal of Medical Internet Research,* 8(2), e9. doi:10.2196/jmir.8.2.e9

Quinn S, Bond R, Nugent C 2017. Quantifying health literacy and ehealth literacy using existing instruments and browser-based software for tracking online health information seeking behavior. *Computers in Human Behavior,* 69, 256–267. doi:10.1016/j.chb.2016.12.032

Sieck CJ, Sheon A, Ancker JS, Castek J, Callahan B, et al. 2021. Digital inclusion as a social determinant of health. *NPJ Digital Medicine,* 4, 52. doi:10.1038/s41746-021-00413-8

Further reading

Broderick J, Devine T, Langhans E, Lemerise AJ, Lier S, et al. 2014. Designing health literate mobile apps. NAM Perspectives. Discussion Paper, National Academy of Medicine, Washington, DC. doi:10.31478/201401a

Kim H, Xie B 2017. Health literacy in the eHealth era: a systematic review of the literature. *Patient Education and Counseling,* 100(6), 1073–1082. doi:10.1016/j.pec.2017.01.015.

McCool J, Dobson R, Whittaker R, Paton C 2022. Mobile health (mHealth) in low- and middle-income countries. *Annual Review of Public Health,* 43, 525–39. doi:10.1146/annurev-publhealth-052620-093850

Nordheim LV, Gundersen MW, Espehaug B, Guttersrud Ø, Flottorp S 2016. Effects of school-based educational interventions for enhancing adolescents' abilities in critical appraisal of health claims: a systematic review. *PLOS One,* 11(8), e0161485-e0161485. doi:10.1371/journal.pone.0161485

Pourrazavi S, Kouzekanani K, Bazargan-Hejazi S, et al. 2020. Theory-based E-health literacy interventions in older adults: a systematic review. *Archives of Public Health,* 78(1), 72. doi:10.1186/s13690-020-00455-6

Rubinelli S, Purnat TD, Wilhelm E, Traicoff D, Namageyo-Funa A, et al. 2022. WHO competency framework for health authorities and institutions to manage infodemics: its development and features. *Human Resources for Health,* 20(1), 35. doi:10.1186/s12960-022-00733-0

Suarez-Lledo V, Alvarez-Galvez J 2021. Prevalence of health misinformation on social media: systematic review. *Journal of Medical Internet Research,* 23(1), e17187. doi:10.2196/17187.

Swire-Thompson B, Lazer D 2020. Public health and online misinformation: challenges and recommendations. *Annual Review of Public Health,* 41(1), 433–451. doi:10.1146/annurev-publhealth-040119-094127

Useful websites

Health Literacy Online: https://health.gov/healthliteracyonline/

Trust It or Trash It: http://www.trustortrash.org

WHO "Mythbusters" infographic series: https://www.who.int/emergencies/ diseases/novel-coronavirus-2019/advice-for-public/myth-busters

WHO online infodemic training: https://openwho.org/courses/infodemic-management-101

5

Health-literate systems and organisations

5.1 Introduction

In Chapter 4, we considered the health literacy opportunities and challenges provided by digital communication platforms. While we explored the distinctive health literacy skills described as eHealth literacy, the focus of the chapter was on how we create information access and utility for those seeking health information online—reducing system complexity more than developing individual health literacy skills. This chapter continues in this direction by examining health literacy at an organisational level.

Most existing national health literacy policies and strategies recognise that the responsiveness of the health system to variations in the health literacy of patients needs to be improved. These make clear that organisational change is required, with the necessary action expressed in different forms, such as "embedding health literacy into systems" and "promoting changes in the healthcare system". Though most attention has been given to the health system, the strategy to reduce organisational complexity can be applied to other organisations and settings, such as schools.

In this chapter, we focus on this concept of "organisational health literacy", identifying relevant models and frameworks as well as examples of current best practice.

5.2 Characteristics of health-literate organisations

Healthcare organisations, their frontline health professionals and health services administrators all play a major role in building, promoting and sustaining health literacy for patients and caregivers. Systematically addressing health literacy at an organisational level has the potential to deliver a range of benefits in higher healthcare quality, reduced costs and improved health outcomes.

"Organisational health literacy" has been defined as "an organisation-wide effort to transform the organisation's delivery of care and services to make it easier for people to navigate, understand and use information and services to take care of their health" (Brach, 2017).

Over the past 20 years considerable attention has been given to the translation of the concept of a health-literate organisation into a set of well-defined and measurable attributes. This has been backed by the development of practical tools and, increasingly, by real-world experience with implementation.

In the US, the Institute of Medicine (IOM) has identified 10 attributes of health-literate organisations, including, for example, leadership that makes health literacy integral to its mission, structure and operations; an engaged and well-trained workforce; co-design; implementation and evaluation of health information and services; and the distribution of print, audio-visual and social media content that is easy to understand and act on. Although this listing of attributes was designed with US healthcare organisations in mind, it has wider applicability to most healthcare organisations. The Australian Commission on Safety and Quality in Health Care (ACSQHC), for example, has used this framework to identify practical actions that health organisations, such as hospitals and clinics, can take as a response to these attributes. Table 5.1 combines information from both sources to provide a comprehensive checklist for use in assessment, action and monitoring activities to promote health-literate organisations.

5.3 Managing change in health organisations

A range of strategies has been proposed to help create health-literate organisations. These are intended to reduce the demands and complexities faced by people engaging with healthcare institutions and health professionals. Not all organisations will be in a position to take action on all 10 of the attributes listed in Table 5.1 at one time, but this list does highlight some essential features and potential approaches to achieving change in health organisations.

Table 5.1 Attributes of health-literate health service organisations

Attribute	Examples of actions that can be taken by organisations
1. Visible leadership: Has leadership that makes health literacy integral to the mission, structure and operations of the healthcare organisation	■ Assign responsibility to an individual or group for actions to improve the health literacy environment ■ Design the physical environment to support effective communication and navigation ■ Make clear and effective communication a priority across all levels of the organisation and all communication channels

(Continued)

Attribute	Examples of actions that can be taken by organisations
2. System-wide integration: Integrates health literacy into planning, evaluation measures, patient safety and quality improvement	■ Audit the health literacy environment (either in the annual audit program of the healthcare organisation or by running a stand-alone audit) ■ Ensure that safety and quality and other improvement initiatives reflect health literacy principles and are evaluated to ensure that they improve the health literacy environment ■ Align a focus on health literacy with other organisational priorities, such as reducing health disparities and providing patient-centred care
3. Trained workforce: Prepares the workforce to be health literate, and monitors progress	■ Incorporate health literacy into orientation sessions and other types of training for the workforce ■ Provide training that highlights the importance of health literacy and strategies to reduce barriers for administrative and front-of-house staff, such as receptionists
4. Consumer co-designed: Includes populations served by the organisation in the design, implementation and evaluation of health information and services	■ Involve consumers in governance processes ■ Collaborate with members of the target community in the design and testing of interventions, including design of facilities, redesign projects and evaluation
5. Universal precautions: Meets the needs of populations with a range of health literacy skills while avoiding stigmatisation	■ Adopt an approach to health literacy that does not make assumptions about levels of individual health literacy (the universal precautions approach) ■ Provide alternatives to written information where possible, and create an environment that does not impose high literacy demands (such as walls and bulletin boards that are not covered with a lot of print information)
6. Effective communication: Uses health literacy strategies in interpersonal communication, and confirms understanding at all points of contact	■ Foster a culture that emphasises verification of understanding of every communication (both clinical and non-clinical) ■ Plan for and provide language assistance where needed, and treat communication failures as patient safety issues

(Continued)

Table 5.1 (*Continued*)

Attribute	Examples of actions that can be taken by organisations
7. Accessible and navigable: Provides easy access to health information and services, and navigation assistance	■ Building design and features that help people find their way to the services they need ■ Use easily understood language and symbols on signage ■ Ensure that information that is available about local resources and services can be understood by consumers with low levels of literacy
8. High utility: Designs and distributes print, audio-visual and social media content that is easy to understand and act on	■ Stock high-quality educational materials that are appropriate for consumers with low health literacy ■ Choose materials that reflect health literacy principles ■ Test consumer information publications as part of the development process with the target audience through surveys, focus groups or other engagement strategies
9. Targeted to risk and need: Addresses health literacy in high-risk situations, including care transitions and information about medicines	■ Identify high-risk situations and establish plans to ensure safe communication in areas such as informed consent, referrals, end-of-life care or use of medicines
10. Customised to system: Communicates clearly about what is covered by public health services and private plans and what individuals will have to pay for services	■ Provide easy-to-understand descriptions of healthcare rights and responsibilities, and communicate the out-of-pocket costs for healthcare services before they are delivered

Source: Australian Commission on Safety and Quality in Health Care 2014. Health literacy: Taking action to improve safety and quality. © Commonwealth of Australia. https://www.safetyandquality. gov.au/sites/default/files/migrated/Health-Literacy-Taking-action-to-improve-safety-and-quality.pdf

Most of our understanding of how to produce organisational change has come from management theory (and practice). This body of theory and knowledge has developed to explain organisational change for a variety of purposes, often in relation to improving organisational performance. There are some helpful reviews of organisational change theory applied to health promotion listed in the further reading at the end of the chapter. These identify different models of change, including stage theory, organisational development theory and diffusion of innovation theory. Stage theory offers a practical approach to change in organisations that includes important elements of these different approaches across four stages of organisational change. These are considered as follows.

Awareness raising

Senior management commitment is essential to achieve sustainable change. Senior individuals act as gatekeepers and are likely to be the most influential in decisions to adopt new policies and programs in an organisation. Those of us who want to see more health-literate organisations have a role in advocating to individuals in leadership roles the benefits from evidence indicating improved patient safety and healthcare quality, cost savings and improved health outcomes.

This advocacy process will be more compelling if it also identifies the parts of the organisation and the key people who would need to be involved in bringing about change. Describing the problem *and* the solution is key. This can be enabled by organisational self-assessments and/or environmental scans to identify where organisational health literacy needs to be improved— for example, by using an organisational health literacy checklist. There are many of these checklists available. Some are very comprehensive and time-consuming and may not be fit for the purpose you have in mind. You should consider carefully which might be best for you by focusing on those developed in your country (where available) or for similar healthcare systems. It may also be practical to examine those domains that you consider most amenable to change in the short term if the full assessment is too demanding. This can help build confidence with senior managers that change is necessary and feasible. Examples are included in the references at the end of this chapter.

At this early stage in the process, senior managers will need assurance that your proposals for change do not cause undue disruption to the core business of the organisation and that the level of resources required is proportionate to the perceived benefits. Getting senior individuals engaged with your proposal and identifying the organisational facilitators and barriers enables you to "unfreeze" the organisation and move to the next stage.

To enable this process, some countries, most notably Australia, have incorporated features of health-literate organisations into regulations governing the accreditation of healthcare organisations—ensuring that there is system-wide verification of progress in improving the quality of health information and communication in health organisations, and structured consumer involvement in healthcare. This regulatory requirement has provided a necessary prompt to senior administrators to engage with the issue and helps to keep some of the key elements of the framework for health-literate organisations front of mind. Other countries may have similar requirements linked to healthcare safety and quality that could be similarly utilised.

Adoption

This stage involves planning for and the adoption of a policy, program or other innovation that addresses the problem identified in Stage 1, including securing the resources (internal and external) necessary for implementation. The type of organisational health literacy self-assessments referred to help us identify which parts of an organisation (structures, resources, people and policies) are critical to change and how to facilitate alignment with the adoption and implementation of an intervention. Staff need to be well informed and prepared to contribute to the implementation of innovation.

Organisations have different cultures and "climates" that influence the feasibility of introducing change and innovation. Introducing change in larger and more complex organisations, such as hospitals, may best be done incrementally—working with the willing to demonstrate feasibility of change and the achievement of benefits. This can be helpfully underpinned by local policies and regulations (see Case study 5.1) as well as the regulatory requirements such as those needed for accreditation (referred to earlier).

Implementation and scale-up

Having identified willing partners in introducing change, it is important that staff feel confident about making change and have the support necessary to do so. This can include staff training and the provision of improved communication resources. This capacity building is essential for the successful introduction and maintenance of change. Little progress will be achieved without staff engagement. Surveys indicate that there is surprisingly low staff awareness of health literacy, its impact on healthcare safety and quality, and ways in which this can be addressed (Cafiero, 2013). Chapter 2 makes clear that there are a range of practical actions that frontline health professionals can take to adopt universal precautions to address health literacy in clinical practice. These require both training and a culture within routine clinical practice that supports excellent communication with patients and caregivers. There are good examples of how this training can be organised and a wide range of training tools and support materials that can be used. For example, Kaper et al. (2019) developed and evaluated a training model successfully used in three countries in Europe to improve confidence and skills in health communication of frontline health practitioners. Table 5.2 provides a summary of the five key learning objectives and related content.

Consideration of training needs should incorporate opportunities in pre-registration education as well as in-service education.

Table 5.2 Overview of Kaper et al.'s (2019) Health Literacy Communication Training program

Session	Learning objectives	Contents
1. Evidence informed knowledge of health literacy (2 h).	A. To inform and educate: Professionals know about health literacy problems, and interventions to tackle health literacy problems.	Identify limited health literacy skills of patients: ▪ Define functional, interactive and critical health literacy. ▪ Discuss the consequences, prevalence and impact of limited health literacy on patients. ▪ Assess written education materials for limited health literacy. ▪ Describe cues and questions to identify health literacy.
2. Gathering and providing information to address functional health literacy (1.5 h).	B. To teach skills: Professionals develop patient-centred communication skills to address problems with health literacy.	Demonstrate skills to gather and provide information: ▪ Gather information by active listening, open questions, establish health literacy level, observe non-verbal signs, and explore emotions and potential feelings of shame. ▪ Provide and prioritise information, use plain language, speak slowly, verify with teach-back if patients understand information.
3. Shared decision-making to address interactive health literacy (1.5 h).	as above	Demonstrate shared decision-making skills: ▪ Invite patients into shared decision-making and make them aware they have a choice. ▪ Facilitate and educate patients to participate in decision-making if needed; i.e. how to disclose their concerns, ask questions and state their preferences. ▪ Explain options; provide comprehensible information relating to prior knowledge. Discuss harms and benefits. ▪ Involve the patient in decision-making; consider pros and cons and individual considerations.

(Continued)

Table 5.2 (Continued)

Session	Learning objectives	Contents
4. Self-management to enhance critical health literacy (1.5 h).	as above	Demonstrate skills to enable self-management: ■ Discuss how to prepare for self-management. ■ Explore patient's readiness for behaviour change and barriers to adherence. ■ Incorporate patient's perspective to enable self-management; formulate personal goals and strengthen self-efficacy. ■ Provide realistic instructions tailored to prior knowledge of patients and their living situation. ■ Discuss required follow-up: monitor self-care, review information and arrangement of support.
5. Applying and sustaining health literacy communication (1.5 h).	C. To support behaviour change: Professionals adopt, change and maintain behaviour to address health literacy problems.	Demonstrate sustainable application of health literacy communication skills into practice: ■ Discuss and share experiences on application of health literacy communication. ■ Develop a practical tool or action plan to sustain communication in daily practice.

Source: Kaper, M.S., Winter, A.F.D., Bevilacqua, R., Giammarchi, C., McCusker, A., Sixsmith, J; Koot, J.A.R., & Reijneveld, S.A. (2019) Positive outcomes of a comprehensive health literacy communication training for health professionals in three european countries: a multi-centre pre-post intervention study. International Journal of Environmental Research and Public Health, 16, 3923. doi:10.3390/ijerph16203923

Both organisational climate and culture can influence an organisation's capacity to function effectively, and in turn may determine the outcome of efforts to bring about change. More substantial and sustainable change will only be feasible if sufficient attention has been given to the earlier phases of awareness and adoption, with close attention being paid to the fit with the core business of the organisation.

Institutionalising the change—refreezing the system

This final stage is concerned with the long-term maintenance of change. Experience has taught us that progressive implementation of an intervention does not necessarily lead to sustained change. At this stage, those in leadership positions have significant roles in reinforcing and rewarding the changes to "refreeze" the practical changes that have been introduced, and to embed these in changes in the organisation's culture and climate. This can be greatly assisted by change to the physical environment and system-wide support for staff.

Physical change may be reflected in action to ensure that health services are easily navigable and accessible for patients and visitors, and that all forms of routine communication intended for use by the general public fit with the health literacy needs of the patient population. These are practical changes that can have a very positive impact on the experience of patients and the long-term success of their treatment and care. These include:

■ well-designed appointment forms and discharge instructions;
■ clear wayfinding, especially in larger facilities;
■ standardised templates for providing patient information; and
■ health literacy quality control procedures that bring improvements into "business as usual".

There are a small but increasing number of examples of health organisations introducing systems that are designed to raise standards of communication and sustain change. One of these is presented in Case study 5.1.

The literature on organisational change is vast and can be overwhelming. In this section, we have used one of the less complex models to describe organisational change in stages. This model can be used to provide structure to an intervention to improve organisational health literacy by prompting careful consideration of the key processes of change and their sequencing. The four-stage model is helpful in illustrating the need for an incremental approach to changing organisations through structures and people. It is particularly helpful in illustrating the ways in which organisations function at different levels, and how each stage may require involvement of different levels (senior and middle managers, frontline staff).

The delivery of effective, timely and quality organisational change to address health literacy will only be possible and sustainable by working

CASE STUDY 5.1: Creating a health literacy organisational support system in regional New South Wales, Australia

The Illawarra Shoalhaven Local Health District (the Health District) is a regional health service located in NSW, Australia, comprising nine hospitals and with a resident population of approximately 390,000 people. Over a period of 3 years, the Health District implemented a series of organisational changes to improve health literacy. The process broadly followed the four stages of organisational change described in the text.

1. **Awareness raising**: Awareness among the local health executive of the importance of health literacy and its link with quality and safety within the healthcare service initially came about by two "clinical incidents" in the Health District. The first of these followed an enquiry into the death of a patient following routine elective surgery which recommended discharge instructions include information about the signs and symptoms of potential complications in plain English. The second was a quality improvement project which identified that 40% of elective surgery cancellations were due to miscommunication with patients, notably a failure to fast. These incidents reinforced the need for system-wide attention to communication quality within the health district. Senior executives also recognised that a coordinated approach to address health literacy was important to meet the new National Safety and Quality Health Service Standards and accreditation requirements for the organisation.

   During the same period, the Health District also recorded a large number of consumer experience stories. Consumers consistently reported difficulties with access to information, navigating the healthcare system and communicating with providers. These tangible examples of local consumer experiences complemented the initial impetus provided by improvements to clinical safety and quality, and helped shape the District's organisational health literacy approach and initial areas of focus.

2. **Adoption**: The Health District created a health literacy portfolio from within its existing resources. Responsibilities of the health literacy portfolio included consultation with managers, clinicians and consumers to develop and implement a Health Literacy Framework and provide support to facilitate health literacy improvement initiatives in health services across the district.

(Continued)

The Framework incorporated elements from both the US Institute of Medicine's "Ten Attributes of Health Literate Health Care Organizations" and the World Health Organization's "Framework for Action on Health Systems" and included key elements of organisational change. A core component of the Framework was a coordinated, whole-of-organisation system with standardised processes and tools for staff to prepare, review and store plain-language, locally developed, written patient information.

3. **Implementation and scale-up:** To facilitate implementation and scale-up of health literacy practices related to the development of written patient information, an interactive intranet site was developed and a Patient Information Coordinator who managed the process and supported staff to develop resources was appointed. Governance structures were put in place to require staff to use the standardised processes to develop patient information and education materials, as was a Health Literacy Ambassador program which trained staff to be health literacy champions and lead their teams in developing plain-language materials across the district.

4. **Institutionalising the change—refreezing the system:** Health literacy continues to be considered a quality and safety issue in the Health District. The district is developing indicators to monitor organisational improvements that result from health literacy actions, and early evaluations have shown improvements in understandability and actionability of information across the district. Linking engagement in health literacy endeavours by senior executives to their key performance indicators is another potential mechanism being considered to ensure refreezing of the system.

Source: Vellar, L., Mastroianni, F., & Lambert, K. (2017). Embedding health literacy into health systems: a case study of a regional health service. Australian Health Review, 41(6), 621–625. doi:10.1071/AH16109

together with patients, consumers and their families and carers. As indicated in Case study 5.1, a strong consumer voice complements organisational concerns with clinical quality and safety. Partnering with consumers identifies health communication challenges and blind-spots and helps identify solutions that closely match consumer needs. This partnering with consumers has been shown to result in improved outcomes for healthcare, service delivery, policy and health education. There are a number of ways to engage consumers, with levels of involvement often mapped in the form of a continuum. The International Association for Public Participation, for example, provides a Spectrum of Public Participation which ranges from a 'passive' commitment to inform, through involvement and collaboration to 'empowerment', where there is an overt commitment to make decisions on the basis of full and equal consumer participation. The IAPC Spectrum of Public Participation can be accessed from: https://www.iap2.org.

The level of commitment to public participation described in the IAPC Spectrum will vary for every organisation and issue. It will depend on practical feasibility, as well as the goals, timeframes, resources as well as varying levels of community concern/interest in the process, issue or decision to be made. Regardless, it is important that working relationships with consumers and communities are built on transparent and accountable processes, clear and open communication and wherever feasible, shared goals.

Finally, to get the best outcomes, it is important to involve consumers with a diverse range of backgrounds and perspectives, including varying levels of health literacy. This will increase the chance that organisational changes truly reflect broad consumer and community needs. Achieving this will require that staff have the necessary skills and training to effectively engage and involve consumers. This could include, for example, training in strategies for effective communication outlined in Chapter 2. Simultaneously, consumers should also have access to the resources, induction, training and support they need. By providing the right training for consumers and health organisation staff, and putting in place the right strategies to engage with a broad cross section of consumers, you are helping to set up your organisation for successful and sustainable engagement.

5.4 Extending beyond health organisations

While the great majority of experience in creating health-literate organisations has been with healthcare organisations, some researchers and practitioners have explored other organisations and settings that might be responsive to the concept, especially community service and educational organisations. For example, one of the organisational health literacy checklists provided in the Useful websites at the end of this chapter comes from a community services support organisation, the Tasmanian Council of Social Services, and is in turn a part of a wider community coalition to promote literacy and numeracy in Tasmania that involves a broad range of public and private organisations. This and other examples provide confidence that the concept of a health-literate organisation can be extended beyond the healthcare system into a much broader range of organisational settings and could be incorporated into comprehensive workplace health and safety strategies. Some countries, notably

Germany and Austria, are exploring these possibilities. As is the case with health organisations, change to becoming a more health-literate organisation will depend on our ability to demonstrate a clear fit with "core business", and positive benefit relative to cost, especially outside of the more traditional human services organisations. More research and practical experience are needed to guide progress.

One obvious setting where the fit with core business can most easily be demonstrated is in schools. There is some limited experience with embedding the idea of a school as a health-literate organisation into broader interventions to create health promoting schools. Again, practical experience is limited at present.

5.5 Summary

Health systems are complex and health organisations often operate in ways that make it difficult for people to find the information and healthcare services they need. Becoming a health-literate organisation requires significant, concurrent and multiple changes that require careful coordination and execution. Fortunately, there are some excellent models and practical tools that make progress more achievable. The widely adopted *10 attributes of health-literate organisations* provides a clear framework for the changes needed in health (and other) organisations, and there is growing practical experience in both managing and sustaining change in health organisations. These tools and experiences provide useful guidance on the different steps required to introduce and sustain a change program in organisations. In particular, they highlight:

- **fit with core business:** the need to understand the core business of an organisation, and its organisational structure, to determine how a health-literate organisation can be best fitted within these parameters;
- **action at different levels in the organisation:** the need to work with individuals at different levels in an organisation at different times to get "buy-in" for a health-literate organisation;
- **engagement with gatekeepers:** the importance of flexibility in negotiation with "gatekeepers" concerning the adoption of activities that are not currently part of routine business;
- **capacity-building with staff:** the need to develop capacity among those individuals responsible for the delivery of a program or innovation, especially to equip frontline workers with the skills they need in a health-literate organisation; and
- **a system-wide solution:** the need to understand and engage at a system level to deliver more sophisticated, complete and enduring change.

References

Australian Commission on Safety and Quality in Health Care 2014. *Health literacy: Taking action to improve safety and quality.* Commonwealth of Australia.

Brach C 2017. The journey to become a health literate organization: a snapshot of health system improvement. *Studies in Health Technologies and Informatics,* 240, 203–237.

Cafiero M 2013. Nurse practitioners' knowledge, experience, and intention to use health literacy strategies in clinical practice. *Journal of Health Communication,* 18, 70–81. doi:10.1080/10810730.2013.825665

International Association for Public Participation, https://www.iap2.org/mpage/Home

Kaper MS, Winter AFD, Bevilacqua R, Giammarchi C, McCusker A, et al. 2019. Positive outcomes of a comprehensive health literacy communication training for health professionals in three European countries: a multi-centre pre-post intervention study. *International Journal of Environmental Research and Public Health,* 16, 3923. doi:10.3390/ijerph16203923

Vellar L, Mastroianni F, Lambert K 2017. Embedding health literacy into health systems: a case study of a regional health service. *Australian Health Review,* 41(6), 621–625. doi:10.1071/AH16109

Further reading

Batras D, Duff C, Smith BJ 2016. Organizational change theory: implications for health promotion practice. *Health Promotion International,* 31(1), 231–241. doi:10.1093/heapro/dau098

Butterfoss FD, Kegler MC, Francisco VT 2008. Mobilizing organizations for health promotion: theories of organizational change. In Glanz K, Rimer BK, Viswanath K (eds.), *Health Behavior and Health Education: theory, research, and practice* (pp. 335–361). Jossey-Bass.

Farmanova E, Bonneville L, Bouchard L 2018. Organizational health literacy: review of theories, frameworks, guides, and implementation issues. *INQUIRY: The Journal of Health Care Organization, Provision and Financing,* 55, 46958018757848. doi:10.1177/0046958018757848

Kirchhoff S, Okan O 2022. Health literate schools: organizational health literacy in the school setting. *European Journal of Public Health,* 32(3). doi:10.1093/eurpub/ckac129.249

Rathmann K, Salewski LD, Zelfl LV 2022. Organizational health literacy and health promotion in health care settings: results from Germany. *European Journal of Public Health,* 32(3). doi:10.1093/eurpub/ckac131.360

Sentell T, Foss-Durant A, Patil U, Taira D, Paasche-Orlow MK, et al. 2021. Organizational health literacy: opportunities for patient-centered care in the wake of COVID-19. *Quality Management in Health Care,* 30(1), 49–60. doi:10.1097/QMH.0000000000000279

Useful websites

Enliven Organisational Health Literacy Self-Assessment: https://enliven.org. au/health-literacy-resources/

Health Literacy Environment of Hospitals and Health Centres (HLEHHC) (2): https://cdn1.sph.harvard.edu/wp-content/uploads/sites/135/2019/05/ april-30-FINAL_The-Health-Literacy-Environment2_Locked.pdf

Health Literacy Universal Precautions Toolkit (and the Primary Care Health Literacy Assessment): https://www.ahrq.gov/sites/default/files/ publications/files/healthlittoolkit2_4.pdf

Health Literate Health Care Organization 10 item Questionnaire (HLHO-10): https://bmchealthservres.biomedcentral.com/articles/10.1186/s12913-015-0707-5

HeLLO Tas! Toolkit: https://www.hellotas.org.au/sites/default/files/files/ HeLLOTas%20Toolkit_0.pdf

New Zealand Ministry of Health Health Literacy Review: https://www. health.govt.nz/system/files/documents/publications/health-literacy-review-a-guide-may15-v2.pdf

Organisational Health Literacy Responsiveness (Org-HLR) Self-Assessment Tool: https://www.cec.health.nsw.gov.au/__data/assets/ pdf_file/0007/488095/Trezona-et-al-2018_The-Organisational-Health-Literacy-Responsiveness-self-ax-tool-user-guide.pdf

Vienna Concept of Health-Literate Hospitals and Healthcare Organisations (V-HLO-I): https://bmchealthservres.biomedcentral.com/articles/10.1186/ s12913-021-06211-y

6

Measurement and monitoring in health literacy

6.1 Introduction

In previous chapters we have explored the different ways in which health literacy has been defined and operationalised in clinical, community and organisational settings. In each chapter we have provided case studies and other references reporting on research that has helped us to understand how to work effectively with patients and consumers, community groups and organisations to improve health literacy and/or minimise the impact of poor health literacy. In most cases, this research has involved the measurement of health literacy among individuals and population groups.

Over the past 30 years, several tools have been developed to measure health literacy. Some of these are intended for general use among all types of populations, while others have been developed for more specific purposes and contexts. Like all measurement tools, each has strengths and limitations. In this chapter, we provide an overview of these health literacy measurement tools as well as additional methods for monitoring and evaluation, with an emphasis on their application and utility in different settings.

6.2 Why measure health literacy?

Before deciding on a measurement approach or instrument, it is necessary to consider the purposes of measurement in your circumstances. Being clear about purpose will help you to weigh up the strengths and limitations of different measures and approaches that are discussed later in this chapter.

One common reason for measuring health literacy is to provide an estimate of the proportion of the population within a specific geographical area, health region or health facility that have higher or lower health literacy. Once we have a useable measure of health literacy in a population, we are in a position to identify the personal and social characteristics most associated with higher and lower levels of health literacy (such as age, gender, ethnicity, education and employment status) and explore these relationships. We can also examine the relationship between higher and lower health literacy and health outcomes. This information can then inform subsequent decisions, such as where to concentrate actions and resources. For example, measuring health literacy in clinical settings can help us to determine optimal approaches to written and verbal communication with different patients, and indicate ways to modify services to improve accessibility.

In circumstances where we are engaged in proactive communication and education designed to improve specific health knowledge, skills and competencies, health literacy measurements can be used to evaluate the impact of these interventions (or other actions and policy changes). This would typically involve using a valid health literacy measurement tool with the target population before and after an intervention so that change in knowledge, skills and competencies can be reliably observed.

The focus in this chapter is on measurement, and not on evaluation methods. For more information on the science of evaluation design and methods, please refer to the companion volume to this book *Evaluation in a Nutshell: a practical guide to the evaluation of health promotion programs* (Bauman & Nutbeam, 2022).

6.3 Types of health literacy measures

Decades of research have led to the design and testing of numerous measures of health literacy. The sheer volume of options can be overwhelming when considering what might be most practical for use in specific circumstances. To help navigate this complexity, these measures can be categorised to help identify the type of measurement that is most relevant and practical to use in different circumstances. Figure 6.1 provides a summary classification of the different measures and is explained further.

Format

Firstly, in terms of format, measures of health literacy are categorised as "performance-based" or "self-reported". Performance-based measures (sometimes referred to as "objective" measures) are a direct test of a person's skills.

Figure 6.1 Summary classification of different measures of health literacy

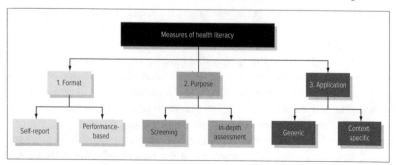

They require a person to complete a task or set of tasks related to their health and then an independent and structured assessment is made on how well they performed these practical tasks. By contrast, self-reported measures are more subjective. People provide answers to carefully constructed questions intended to assess different aspects of their health literacy. They involve individuals providing information (through a questionnaire or interview) that describes themselves and their preferences or skills in ways that cannot be independently verified.

Both performance-based and self-report measures have strengths and weaknesses. Directly measuring a person's performance is inherently more objective. But it can be time consuming, expensive (especially when using more comprehensive measures) and stigmatising for individuals, the majority of whom have difficulty with the tasks required of them. Existing performance-based measures are generally limited in their capacity to assess change over time. By contrast, self-reporting offers greater ease of testing and lower cost in larger surveys, and is less likely to cause embarrassment to the person completing the questionnaire. Self-completion questionnaires are generally more easily adapted for application in a wide range of situations, where there are limitations on the time and support available for administration, and where English-language proficiency is limited and/or translation is required. Multidimensional self-report instruments more closely reflect the type and variety of health literacy skills that are developed during interventions and are more useful than performance-based measures for piloting, revising and evaluating the effectiveness of health literacy interventions.

Performance-based measures of health literacy

Early research and practice in health literacy were dominated by two performance-based measures: the Rapid Estimate of Adult Literacy in Medicine (REALM) and the Short Test of Functional Health Literacy in Adults (S-TOFHLA). The REALM measures a patient's ability to pronounce 66 common medical words and lay terms for body parts and illnesses. The S-TOFHLA tests a person's ability to read passages using real materials from the healthcare setting. As research and understanding of health literacy have evolved over time, these "legacy tools" are less frequently used as they capture only a narrow range of literacy skills.

Other performance-based measures of health literacy have evolved to include a broader range of skills-based questions which require people to demonstrate their understanding and interpretation of health-related information. One of the most commonly used is the Newest Vital Sign (NVS), which is based on a standardised Nutrition Facts label and six accompanying questions, requiring basic reading and numeracy skills (e.g. *"If you eat the entire container, how many calories will you eat?*"). Although focused on nutrition information, the conceptual and analytic skills needed to understand a nutrition label are similar to those needed to respond to most health-related instructions. Figure 6.2 provides an illustration of the original NVS nutrition label and questions. Several adaptations of this have been used in different countries.

Other performance-based health literacy instruments place even greater emphasis on a variety of applied skills. The Health Literacy Skills Instrument (HLSI) (available in short or long form), for example, was designed to measure the ability of users to read and understand text and to locate and interpret information in documents (print literacy), to use quantitative information (numeracy), to listen effectively (oral literacy) and to seek information through the internet (navigation). It includes a range of tasks using a hospital map, medicine record, nutrition label and medical centre audio recording to test skills. Compared to the NVS, this type of instrument assesses a more comprehensive range of literacy skills but inevitably takes longer to administer and analyse. Making a judgment call on which type of instrument is more useful for you will depend on whether you need a quick and reliable measure (such as in clinical practice) or a comprehensive measure that allows for more sophisticated understanding of different health literacy skills (which may be more important for research purposes).

Figure 6.2 Newest Vital Sign

Nutrition Facts	
Serving Size	1/2 cup
Servings per container	4
Amount per serving	
Calories 250	Fat Cal 120
	%DV
Total Fat 13g	20%
Sat Fat 9g	40%
Cholesterol 28mg	12%
Sodium 55mg	2%
Total Carbohydrate 30g	12%
Dietary Fiber 2g	
Sugars 23g	
Protein 4g	8%

* Percent Daily Values (DV) are based on a 2,000 calorie diet. Your daily values may be higher or lower depending on your calorie needs.

Ingredients: Cream, Skim Milk, Liquid Sugar, Water, Egg Yolks, Brown Sugar, Milkfat, Peanut Oil, Sugar, Butter, Salt, Carrageenan, Vanilla Extract.

	ANSWER CORRECT? YES	NO
READ TO SUBJECT: This information is on the back of a container of a pint of ice cream.		
QUESTIONS		
1. If you eat the entire container, how many calories will you eat? **Answer** ❑ 1,000 is the only correct answer	____	____
2. If you are allowed to eat 60 g of carbohydrates as a snack, how much ice cream could you have? **Answer** Any of the following is correct: ❑ 1 cup (or any amount up to 1 cup) ❑ Half the container Note: If patient answers "2 servings," ask "How much ice cream would that be if you were to measure it into a bowl?"	____	____
3. Your doctor advises you to reduce the amount of saturated fat in your diet. You usually have 42 g of saturated fat each day, which includes 1 serving of ice cream. If you stop eating ice cream, how many grams of saturated fat would you be consuming each day? **Answer** 33 is the only correct answer	____	____
4. If you usually eat 2500 calories in a day, what percentage of your daily value of calories will you be eating if you eat one serving? **Answer** 10% is the only correct answer	____	____
Pretend that you are allergic to the following substances: Penicillin, peanuts, latex gloves, and bee stings.		
5. Is it safe for you to eat this ice cream? **Answer** ❑ No	____	____
6. (Ask only if the patient responds "no" to question 5): Why not? **Answer** Because it has peanut oil.	____	____
Total Correct	____	

Source: Reproduced with permission from Weiss BD, Mays MZ, Martz W, et al. Quick assessment of literacy in primary care: the newest vital sign. Ann Fam Med. 2005;3(6):514–522.

Self-reported measures of health literacy

Early self-report instruments were designed primarily for screening rather than comprehensively measuring health literacy. The most used instrument is based on three questions shown to be effective for identifying those with below basic health literacy skills (fifth grade level or less):

1. *How often do you have somebody help you read hospital materials?*
2. *How confident are you filling out medical forms by yourself?*
3. *How often do you have problems learning about your medical condition because of difficulty understanding written information?*

Further evaluations concluded that combinations of multiple questions were no more effective in identifying those with low health literacy than question 2 alone (*"How confident are you filling out medical forms by yourself?"*) and this single item question has subsequently been widely applied in both research and practice.

Beyond these simple measures, several multidimensional self-reported measures of health literacy have been developed over the past 15 years, with a view to provide an in-depth assessment of the different dimensions of health literacy. Two of the best developed and most commonly used are:

■ The *Health Literacy Questionnaire (HLQ),* which comprises nine independent scales related to the understanding of, engagement with and use of health services from both an individual and organisational perspective. These include, for example, social support for health, appraisal of health information, ability to actively engage with healthcare providers, navigating the healthcare system and ability to find good health information. In the first part of the questionnaire, people rate how strongly they disagree or agree with a set of statements (e.g. whether they spend a lot of time actively managing their health). In Part 2, people are asked to indicate how difficult or easy they find a set of specified tasks (e.g. find information about health problems, ask healthcare providers questions, confidently fill medical forms). In this way, the HLQ scales provide a reflection of the quality of health and social service provision as well as individuals' skills. The HLQ has been through substantial and well-documented testing and development (see references at the end of the chapter) and has been applied widely in many different countries, settings and populations. It has been used for population surveys, the development of interventions and evaluation of programs. In some examples, researchers and program evaluators have selected only some of the individual domains represented in the full questionnaire to best match the purposes and intended outcomes of individual programs (Osborne et al., 2013).

■ The *European Health Literacy Survey Questionnaire (HLS-EU-Q47)*, which consists of 47 core self-report items across three health domains: healthcare, disease prevention and health promotion. It extends well beyond the clinical domain and offers a more comprehensive measure of health literacy. Table 6.1 provides an overview of the health literacy matrix developed for the questionnaire, showing in greater detail the three domains and the key elements of health literacy (access, understand, appraise and apply health information). In the questionnaire, all items appear in standardised format to assess the difficulty of specific health tasks from "very difficult" to "very easy". Like the HLQ, the development and application of the *HLS-EU-Q47* is well documented and the questionnaire has been used in different countries with different populations. A shorter version of the questionnaire (HLS-Q12) has also been developed and tested for use, and may be more practical for use as a screening tool or in studies exploring the relationship between health literacy and observed health outcomes.

Table 6.1   HLS-EU health literacy matrix

	Access/obtain information relevant to health	Understand information relevant to health	Process/appraise information relevant to health	Apply/use information relevant to health
Healthcare	Ability to access information on medical and clinical issues	Ability to understand medical information and derive meaning	Ability to interpret and evaluate medical information	Ability to make informed decisions on medical issues
Disease prevention	Ability to access information on risk factors for health	Ability to understand information on risk factors and derive meaning	Ability to interpret and evaluate information on risk factors for health	Ability to make informed decisions on risk factors for health
Health promotion	Ability to update oneself on determinants of health in the social and physical environment	Ability to understand information on determinants of health in the social and physical environment and derive meaning	Ability to interpret and evaluate information on health determinants in the social and physical environment	Ability to make informed decisions on health determinants in the social and physical environment

Source: Sørensen, K., Van den Broucke, S., Pelikan, J.M. et al. Measuring health literacy in populations: illuminating the design and development process of the European Health Literacy Survey Questionnaire (HLS-EU-Q). BMC Public Health 13, 948 (2013). https://doi.org/10.1186/1471-2458-13-948

Purpose

Moving beyond format, Figure 6.1 also identifies that measures of health literacy can be applied for different purposes. These vary from using a tool for screening purposes through to a more complex and in-depth assessment of health literacy. Screening instruments are usually brief, easy-to-administer tools for identifying individuals with low health literacy. They have been most often applied in clinical settings to rapidly identify adults with lower health literacy skills. However, they are not as effective for identifying those with moderate or higher levels of health literacy and, by their nature, do not capture the comprehensive range of skills and attributes embodied in current definitions of health literacy. Simple measures can be very useful in clinical practice to identify individuals who may need additional help in understanding and responding to health and clinical information. They are also used in more comprehensive health surveys as a "marker" for health literacy that can be used as a variable in subsequent analysis. In-depth assessment tools provide a more sophisticated assessment of the different dimensions of health literacy. They usually include multiple questions and often assess a spectrum of abilities related to accessing, understanding and using health information and health services.

Application

Finally, Figure 6.1 indicates that health literacy measures can be generic or context-specific. Generic measures of health literacy have been designed for use with a wide range of populations to measure more universal health literacy characteristics. By their nature, such measurement instruments have to be generalisable and capable of use in a wide variety of circumstances, including for use in population surveys.

By contrast, many measurement instruments have been developed to cover more specific content and contexts. In Chapter 1, we discussed health literacy as being "context-specific", recognising that both content and context change through the life-course. Context-specific measures of health literacy differ from generic tools in that they assess skills, knowledge and competencies required in specific contexts, such as for people living with different health conditions or in different age groups, including children, adolescents and older adults, and specialised measures of health literacy such as eHealth literacy (see Chapter 4).

Given that there are now hundreds of health literacy measurement instruments available, we have focused in this chapter on generic instruments which have been widely applied in the field and are applicable across populations and settings. To find a much wider range of instruments that can be used for specific content or contexts, we recommend the Health Literacy Tool Shed, an online database of health literacy measurement tools. The Tool Shed contains basic information about various tools, including their psychometric properties, based on peer-reviewed literature as well as links to access them; see: https://healthliteracy.bu.edu

6.4 Qualitative approaches to measurement

The chapter so far has focused on quantitative measures of health literacy. An alternative approach are qualitative methods, which generally include data in the form of *words* rather than *numbers,* gathered through methods such as interviews and focus groups. Qualitative methods generally enable us to better understand people's beliefs, experiences, attitudes, behaviour and interactions by allowing us to explore in more depth questions of "why?" and "how?". Qualitative methods can provide a more personal understanding of health literacy and the impacts of health literacy interventions from the perspective of a range of stakeholders.

Qualitative research is also especially effective in obtaining culturally specific information about the values, opinions, behaviours, relationships and social contexts of different populations. Case study 6.1 demonstrates this utility. Through the use of qualitative methods, researchers were able to identify and highlight the complexity and contextuality of health literacy for Ngāti Porou and other Indigenous people. This nuanced and contextualised data would have been difficult to capture by quantitative methods alone.

Case study 6.1 illustrates how qualitative methods are especially helpful when used to extend our understanding and better explain observations that emerge from the use of more quantitative measures such as those described in the previous sections. As before, it is important to be clear about your purpose in using qualitative research, and to make a judgment call on the best fit with your knowledge of diverse needs in a population, the resources available and the added benefit of obtaining the type of insights that qualitative research can provide.

CASE STUDY 6.1: Qualitative evaluation of the Cardiovascular Disease Medicines Health Literacy Intervention

The Cardiovascular Disease Medicines Health Literacy Intervention aimed to strengthen patient health literacy knowledge, skills and practices among Indigenous peoples in Aotearoa, Australia and Canada. To evaluate the impact of the intervention in New Zealand, researchers employed a Kaupapa Māori evaluation (KME) approach, including semi-structured qualitative interviews with six patients participating in the intervention and three

(Continued)

health professionals. The evaluation specifically aimed to identify patient and whānau experiences of and satisfaction with the intervention, reports of changes in understanding and behaviour, and how the intervention could be improved for the future.

Qualitative analysis identified that health literacy was primarily nurtured through health practitioner support. Through ongoing whanaungatanga (relationship, kinship, connection) practices, and reciprocal, responsive relationships that entailed active collaboration, shared power, partnership and deliberative engagement, the intervention was considered to be more powerful and influential, with greater potential to support long-term sustainable change in medication use and practices. The qualitative analysis was also able to identify distributed impacts of the intervention within communities, through information and knowledge sharing facilitated by the research nurse who was integral to the intervention.

6.5 Summary

- **Clarity of purpose:** The different methods for health literacy measurement have strengths and weaknesses that make them more or less well suited for different purposes, including screening, intervention activities and surveillance.
- **Screening:** Simple measures (such as the NVS and single item screener) are most practical to use for the purposes of identifying patients and community members who may be at greatest risk of misunderstanding of health information and advice.
- **Surveillance:** More comprehensive measures provide the broader range of data required to understand health literacy strengths and weaknesses in populations and enable more complex and sophisticated analysis of relationships between different attributes of health literacy, and between health literacy and health outcomes. These include both direct measurement and self-report instruments.

- **Evaluation:** Choice of instrument needs to be dictated by the program/intervention being evaluated, ensuring the best fit between the objectives of the intervention and the health literacy attributes measured. Self-reported instruments are generally more adaptable for the purposes of evaluation, and there are many context-specific instruments available.
- **Qualitative research methods** are a useful addition to established survey instruments, providing insight and understanding not easily obtained from these qualitative instruments.

References

Bauman A, Nutbeam D 2022. *Evaluation in a Nutshell: a practical guide to the evaluation of health promotion programs* (3rd edition). Sydney, McGraw Hill Education Australia Pty Ltd.

Carlson T, Moewaka Barnes H, McCreanor T 2019. Health literacy in action: Kaupapa Māori evaluation of a cardiovascular disease medications health literacy intervention. *AlterNative: An International Journal of Indigenous Peoples,* 15(2), 101–110. doi:10.1177/1177180119828050

Osborne RH, Batterham RW, Elsworth GR Hawkins M, Buchbinder R 2013. The grounded psychometric development and initial validation of the Health Literacy Questionnaire (HLQ). *BMC Public Health*, 13, 658. doi:10.1186/1471-2458-13-658

Sørensen K, Van den Broucke S, Pelikan JM, Fullam J, Doyle G, Hawkins M, Buchbinder R 2013. Measuring health literacy in populations: illuminating the design and development process of the European Health Literacy Survey Questionnaire (HLS-EU-Q). *BMC Public Health,* 13, 948. doi:10.1186/1471-2458-13-948

Weiss BD, Mays MZ, Martz W, Castro KM, DeWalt DA, et al. 2005. Quick assessment of literacy in primary care: the newest vital sign. *Annals of Family Medicine,* 3(6), 514–522. doi:10.1370/afm.405

Further reading

Chew LD, Griffin JM, Partin MR, Noorbaloochi S, Grill JP, et al. 2008. Validation of screening questions for limited health literacy in a large VA outpatient population. *Journal of General Internal Medicine,* May 23(5), 561–566. doi:10.1007/s11606-008-0520-5.

Sørensen K, Van den Broucke S, Pelikan JM Fullam J, Doyle G, et al. 2013. Measuring health literacy in populations: illuminating the design and development process of the European Health Literacy Survey Questionnaire (HLS-EU-Q). *BMC Public Health,* 13, 948. doi:10.1186/1471-2458-13-948

7

Health literacy, equity and the social determinants of health

7.1   Introduction

Health literacy has been criticised for focusing on the role of the individual in healthcare and health improvement. This critique emphasises that too little account is taken of the impact of adverse social and economic conditions that are beyond the immediate control of individuals and the limitations these place on individuals in their options to respond to health communication. This includes the impact of our physical environment, access to education, employment, and adequate housing and income. These conditions can significantly limit individuals' abilities and options to respond to health communications intended to protect or improve health. For example, communications that tell people to change the food they eat when "healthier" food is not available at a price they can afford, or provide healthcare advice that is complex and resource intensive. When our communications require responses from people that are beyond their skills and resources, we run a serious risk of "blaming the victim" and perpetuating already existing inequalities in health. Put simply, those who are better educated and have greater access to resources are often best able to respond to health communications and benefit from them. Those with limited resources get left further behind.

Many of our communications are of necessity directed at individuals, are intended to improve personal knowledge and skills, and are directed to facilitate predetermined changes in behaviour. There is nothing inherently wrong with this "functional" approach to health communication. That said, throughout the book we have consistently emphasised that people have different capacities to respond to standardised communication, and that these capacities are significantly influenced by the demands and complexities of the environment in which communication takes place. The concept of universal health literacy precautions referred to in Chapter 2 has emerged from this understanding of health literacy. Adopting universal precautions in health communication together with organisational action to reduce the demands and complexities of our health services can help reduce the risk that our health communications are only effective with a minority of consumers.

So far, so good; universal health literacy precautions can help mitigate "risk", but do little to develop health literacy as a personal and societal "asset". Neither do they engage people in understanding and acting on the determinants of health that constrain their choices and opportunities. These social, economic and environmental conditions have a profound impact on access to the resources (and power) that enable people to exert greater control over their health.

In Chapter 1, we introduced the concept of critical health literacy to describe the most advanced health literacy skills that can be applied to critically analyse, understand and apply information from a wide range of sources. We have examined in subsequent chapters how more advanced health literacy skills can be developed through the use of interactive communication methods and more diverse content. In this chapter, we consider more deeply the relationship between health literacy, the social determinants of health and greater equity in heath. We focus attention on how to optimise the contribution that improved health literacy can make to addressing inequities in health, recognising that this perspective on health literacy is much less well understood and is an emerging area of research and practice.

7.2 Health literacy as a social determinant of health

Health status is fundamentally determined by the conditions in which we are born, grow, live and age. These conditions, described earlier, include the safety and quality of our physical environment, access to education, adequate employment and income. They fundamentally influence our choice of actions and our capacity to engage successfully in society. These conditions are often referred to as the *social determinants of health*. These social determinants are considered alongside individual characteristics and behaviours as the main drivers of health and disease in populations. Improvements in life expectancy in the past century are generally more attributable to improvements to the social determinants (such as better access to education, improved housing, more nutritious foods) than with medical therapies, though both are important.

These social determinants are also considered to be the major drivers of observable inequities in health—put simply, those from more disadvantaged backgrounds generally have poorer health and more constrained opportunities to improve and protect their health. The WHO recognises that addressing the causes and impact of the social determinants of health is the most important route to reducing inequities in health, and has consistently advocated for change, notably through the work of the WHO Commission on the Social Determinants of Health (WHO, 2008).

Most national surveys of health literacy have identified a strong and consistent relationship between health literacy and these social determinants of health. Researchers have sought to better understand this relationship in order to identify what role (if any) health literacy may have in either causing or moderating the impact of these social determinants of health. This work is attempting to throw light on complex causal relationships. Is poor health literacy caused by social disadvantage, or is poor health literacy a cause of social disadvantage? And importantly, if we can improve health literacy in a community, will this provide some protection against social disadvantage?

Our understanding of these relationships continues to evolve. One of the most substantial examinations of the relationships has come from work undertaken as part of the European Health Literacy Survey undertaken in 2011 in eight European countries. This work, and the work of other researchers, has examined the relationship between social determinants, health literacy and health status. This study found the strongest associations between educational attainment (years in formal education, highest qualification) and health literacy. Income, occupation and ethnicity were also consistently associated with health literacy. In summary, these data and other related studies have provided consistent evidence that those who are already socially disadvantaged tend to have poorer health literacy. This observation confirms that there is a relationship between health literacy and social disadvantage, but doesn't explain whether poor health literacy is a cause or consequence of social disadvantage.

Further analysis of the findings from the European study have provided some limited evidence that, for populations in eight European countries, comprehensive health literacy is a "relevant, independent, direct determinant of self-assessed health" (Pelikan et al., 2018). This means that the researchers observed a consistent relationship between health literacy and health outcomes, regardless of the influence of other social determinants.

This and other research have led us to conclude that health literacy can offer a "mediating role" in the relationship between the social determinants of health and observed health outcomes. Specifically, this means that there is a reasonable likelihood that health literacy can offset the association between social disadvantage and specific health outcomes, health-related behaviours, and in access to and use of health services. The reasonable conclusion is that strengthening health literacy in the population offers a practical strategy to promote greater equity in health.

That said, great care should be taken in promoting health literacy as some kind of panacea for wider problems in our communities and societies. While there is undoubtedly some scope to improve health equity through interventions that address low health literacy, this should not be regarded as a substitute for the need to tackle the underlying societal drivers of inequity (access to education, adequate housing, employment and income) and the need to address underlying root causes in the distribution of power, resources and opportunity.

7.3 Targeting communications to priority populations

In each of the chapters of this book we have identified interventions to improve health literacy in clinical and community populations. Several of the interventions we have featured as case studies were designed and delivered to meet the needs of socially disadvantaged populations. These and many other case studies demonstrate the feasibility of tailoring interventions to address specific population risks and need. Most reported interventions to improve health literacy reflect this concept of (low) health literacy as a "risk" that could be better managed through successful interventions to increase consumer access to reliable information and confidence to apply that information in making decisions about their health, alongside systemic actions to reduce the complexity of health communications.

Targeting high-risk populations is a well-established response to identifiable disadvantage in defined communities. For example, during the COVID-19 pandemic it quickly became apparent that generic messaging, while necessary, was not sufficient to reach highly diverse communities with distinctive preferences for media and messaging. Research demonstrated huge variations in knowledge, attitudes and media use among different groups. This led to some highly targeted communication campaigns using differentiated messaging and media to reach multiple cultural and language groups with essential information about COVID-19. These targeted communication campaigns, leveraging research findings and existing community strengths and networks, were far more successful in reaching a broader range of communities, including many that would be classified as socially disadvantaged. Case study 7.1 provides an example of this type of differentiated communication.

CASE STUDY 7.1: Tailoring COVID-19 messaging to meet the needs of diverse populations

Sydney, Australia, has a highly diverse population of almost 5 million residents. Generic messaging on prevention combined with very strict lockdowns had been successful in controlling the first phases of the COVID-19 pandemic prior to the widespread availability of a vaccine. By mid-2021, vaccines had become available in Australia but initial uptake was variable across different population groups. In the period March to July 2021, researchers at the University of Sydney undertook a survey to explore COVID-19 information sources, knowledge, behaviour and vaccine intentions

(Continued)

for people from culturally and linguistically diverse communities. The survey was co-designed with bilingual staff from local health organisations and translated into languages spoken by 11 priority groups in the region.

This detailed local evidence showed that current pandemic communications were not meeting community needs. People who were older, with low health literacy and poor English proficiency had difficulty finding COVID-19 information they could understand. Across the sample, 53% were willing to get a COVID-19 vaccine, though this ranged from 29% to 98%, depending on the language group.

The study also identified that people used a highly diverse range of COVID-19 information sources. For example, people with low health literacy and older people relied heavily on friends or family living in Australia and local community sources. The findings also identified competing information sources; for example, almost one in three participants relied on overseas information sources to learn about COVID-19, with rates ranging from 5% to 98% depending on the language group.

The survey results, together with findings from rapid community consultations conducted by the health organisations, identified that more targeted and community-based approaches to communication were needed. The need for effective communication was heightened as the Delta variant reached Sydney in July 2021, leading to a prolonged lockdown, concurrent with a major drive to improve vaccine uptake. The survey results were immediately made available to the Health Ministry staff responsible for health communications and in all 11 languages to the local health staff working directly with the local communities. This was followed by significant changes to communication plans to develop a series of "micro-strategies" with differentiated communication content and more selective use of media to better target messages to different communities. This was supplemented by provision of translated materials for direct use with local communities by frontline health workers as well as through the use of alternate communication channels, such as trusted advisors (leaders and members of the community), and COVID 19 safety champions who were trained and delivered vaccination sessions in-language or in English, reaching >6000 community members across a diverse range of community groups.

The study provided timely and actionable findings that could be implemented rapidly within the context of the Delta outbreak in diverse communities in Sydney. By mid-September 2021, 84% overall and greater than 95% of adult residents in some of the most disadvantaged communities in Sydney had received their first COVID-19 vaccine dose. This compared

(Continued)

with 82% of the state of New South Wales as a whole. This represents much higher and faster uptake than anticipated, taking into account that only 53% of participants in the original study reported willingness to get the vaccine during the months prior. (Ayre et al.,2022 & Zachariah et al.,2022)

Our experiences with COVID-19 and many other examples shows us that the application of universal health literacy precautions as the basis for generic communications is a necessary step in managing the "risk" associated with low health literacy, but it may not be sufficient to reach those populations most impacted by social disadvantage. Our experience with the pandemic has provided an important reminder that more comprehensive, systemic responses are required to support the improvement of health literacy differentially between and within different population groups.

Such an approach is based on providing "universally accessible" health services and resources (including access to/engagement with health information) with a scale and intensity that is proportionate to the level of disadvantage. Put simply, health literacy interventions should be as accessible, reliable, understandable and usable as possible for everyone in the population, *but* be disproportionately focused on reaching and engaging the population groups most impacted by low health literacy. This is subtly but significantly different to adopting universal precautions, and consolidates the preferential commitment of resources to address the needs of those most disadvantaged. In Case study 7.1, this required greater investment in highly differentiated communications (both media and messaging) to reach priority populations in the community to improve vaccine uptake in some of the most disadvantaged communities. This is often referred to as *proportionate universalism.*

Using this principle of proportionate universalism to guide our investments of time and material resources in health literacy can help manage the risk that we might inadvertently exacerbate existing health inequities. But it does not automatically optimise the potential contribution that improved health literacy could make to reducing inequities. This requires us to work with individuals and communities to build more advanced and transferable skills that are represented in the concept of critical health literacy.

7.4   Improving critical health literacy

Functional health literacy tends to be goal directed, supported by communications that enable access and use of health information to make well-defined decisions about health and healthcare. Our role as communicators is to guide as "experts". The concept of interactive health literacy shifts our focus onto the development of skills that can be adapted to changing circumstances and enable people to interact more successfully with different sources of information, including interactions with health professionals. These skills are "transferable"–not limited to specific information, actions or points in time. They are generic skills in finding, appraising and understanding reliable health information, and skills that foster confidence to act on this information at different times and in different environments. Our role as communicators is more educational as partners in learning, and less as guiding expert. This type of communication generally needs to be more interactive, drawing upon the experience of learners as well as our expertise as communicators.

Critical health literacy differs from functional and interactive health literacy through communication content, purpose and method. Building critical health literacy expands on the generic skills described earlier to include the development of critical appraisal skills and of broader knowledge and understanding of the full range of determinants of health. Table 7.1 provides a useful summary of three domains of critical health literacy and related skills, knowledge and outcomes. These domains helpfully differentiate critical health literacy through its emphasis on skills in critical appraisal of information, understanding of the social determinants of health and recognition of the need for collective action. It also describes extensively some distinctive measurable outcomes associated with critical health literacy, including, for example, skills in social and community organisation, self-advocacy and political action that enable people to have greater influence over a broader range of determinants in health. Our role as communicator is now one of facilitator, advocate and consultant, responding to health priorities that are determined by our consumers and communities. This requires a fundamentally different relationship to the more conventional (and comfortable) relationships we may have as "expert" and "educator".

Experience in working with people to develop critical health literacy is still relatively rare. Most published reviews focus more on the concept and theory than reporting on practical experience (see Abel & Benkert, 2022). One useful review of programs designed for older people identified studies that developed critical health literacy by addressing factors that indirectly influenced older adults' health and wellbeing, including personal and lifestyle factors, cultural conditions and the healthcare system. In this way, these studies "implicitly" addressed older adults' understanding of the social determinants of health. Some of the studies also addressed critical health literacy by focusing on collective actions (de Wit et al., 2017).

De Wit and colleagues' review was also useful in identifying two practices that may contribute to the development of critical health literacy: collaborative learning and social support. Through co-learning (underpinned by mutual respect between "professionals" and community members, and between community members), both community members and health professionals can build critical health

Table 7.1   Domains of critical health literacy

Critical health literacy domain	Skills	Knowledge	Linked concepts	Observable outcomes
Critical appraisal of information	Cognitive skills in managing and interpreting information, including remembering, synthesising, abstracting Reflexivity—assessing personal relevance of information	Scientific methods Medical knowledge	Evidence-based medicine E-literacy Media literacy	Personal research into health Questioning of health information
Understanding social determinants of health	Cognitive skills as above	Health inequalities Social and political structures and realities	Media literacy Conscientisation Empowerment	Changed patterns of consumption Questioning of health information
Collective action	Community organising (planning, goal setting, prioritising) Self-advocacy Communication and personal interaction skills	Health inequalities Social and political structures and realities	Psychological Empowerment Social capital Emancipation	Social action for health Democratic participation

Source: Chinn, D. (2011). Critical Health Literacy: A Review and Critical Analysis. Social science & medicine (1982). 73. 60-7. 10.1016/j.socscimed.2011.04.004.

literacy by learning from each other's experiences and knowledge. Emotional (e.g. sharing experiences), instrumental (e.g. tangible aid), informational (e.g. advice and information), and appraisal (e.g. information for self-evaluation) support can also serve to enhance individuals' critical health literacy.

Beyond this, there is also much that can be learned from established approaches to community building and community mobilisation (Minkler, 2012). These methodologies emphasise the importance of developing community competencies (reflecting organising and advocacy skills) and community control (reflecting the change in relationship between communicator and community). More information on these concepts can be found in the companion volume to this book, *Theory in a Nutshell: a practical guide to health promotion theories* (Nutbeam et al., 2022).

7.5 Summary

Health literacy is a personal and societal asset: By engaging people in understanding and acting on the underlying determinants of health that constrain their choices and opportunities, we can enable people to exert greater control over their health.

Health literacy is not a panacea for health inequities: Health inequities are largely created by the maldistribution of opportunity, resources and power. But it is possible to optimise both the contribution health literacy makes in mediating the causes and effects of inequity, and to empower people to exert greater control over the determinants of health. Strengthening health literacy in the population and making health services more accessible to people with low health literacy can be a practical strategy to promote greater equity in health.

Health literacy interventions should be prioritised for those with greatest need: While the principle of universal precautions remains important, priority should be proportionate to need—our focus has to be on reaching and engaging the population groups disproportionately affected by low health literacy.

Improving critical health literacy can optimise impact on health inequities: Critical health literacy incorporates more comprehensive knowledge of the determinants of health and extended, transferable skills in social organisation, advocacy and political action that enable people to have greater influence over a broader range of determinants in health. The role of the health professional/ communicator is that of facilitator for health priorities and actions that are determined by the consumers and communities themselves.

References

Abel T, Benkert R 2022. Critical health literacy: reflection and action for health. *Health Promotion International,* 37(4). doi:10.1093/heapro/daac114

Ayre J, Muscat DM, Mac O, Batcup C, Cvejic E, et al. 2022. Main COVID-19 information sources in a culturally and linguistically diverse community in Sydney, Australia: a cross-sectional survey. *Patient Education and Counseling,* 105(8): 2793-2800. doi:10.1016/j.pec.2022.03.028

Chinn D 2011. Critical health literacy: a review and critical analysis. *Social Science & Medicine,* 73, 60–67. doi: 10.1016/j.socscimed.2011.04.004

de Wit L, Fenenga C, Giammarchi C, di Furia L, Hutter I, et al. 2018. Community-based initiatives improving critical health literacy: a systematic review and meta-synthesis of qualitative evidence. *BMC Public Health,* 18, 40. doi:10.1186/s12889-017-4570-7

Minkler M (ed) 2012.*Community Organizing and Community Building for Health and Welfare.* New Jersey. Rutgers University Press.

Nutbeam D, Harris E, Wise M 2022. *Theory in a Nutshell: a practical guide to health promotion theories* (4th edition). Sydney, McGraw Hill Education Australia Pty Ltd.

Pelikan JM, Ganahi K, Roethlin F 2018. Health literacy as a determinant, mediator and/or moderator of health: empirical models using the European Health Literacy Survey Data Set. *Global Health Promotion,* 25, 55–66. doi: 10.1177/1757975918788300.

World Health Organization 2008. Closing the gap in a generation: health equity through action on the social determinants of health. Commission on Social Determinants of Health final report. Geneva, Switzerland: World Health Organization, https://apps.who.int/iris/bitstream/handle/10665/43943/9789241563703_eng.pdf

Zachariah D, Mouwad D, Muscat DM, Ayre J, Nutbeam D, et al. 2022. Addressing the health literacy needs and experiences of culturally and linguistically diverse populations in Australia during COVID-19: a research embedded participatory approach. *Journal of Health Communication,* 27(7), 439–449. doi: 10.1080/10810730.2022.2118910

Further reading

Mogford E, Gould L, Devoght A 2011. Teaching critical health literacy in the US as a means to action on the social determinants of health. *Health Promotion International,* 26(1), 4–13. doi:10.1093/heapro/daq049

Nutbeam D, Lloyd JE 2021. Understanding and responding to health literacy as a social determinant of health. *Annual Review of Public Health,* 42(1), 159–173. doi:10.1146/annurev-publhealth-090419-102529

Stormacq C, Van den Broucke S, Wosinski J 2019. Does health literacy mediate the relationship between socioeconomic status and health disparities? Integrative review. *Health Promotion International,* 34, e1–e17. doi:10.1093/heapro/day062

Sykes S, Wills J, Rowlands G, Popple K 2013. Understanding critical health literacy: a concept analysis. *BMC Public Health,* 13(1), 150. doi:10.1186/1471-2458-13-150

index